DATE			
DEC 1 3 2002	JUN 1 8 2003		
DEC 2 6 2002			
JAN 6 2003	JUL -5 2003		
JAN 3 0 2003	DEC 2 2 2003		
FEB 1 3 2003	AUG 1 1 2005		
	AUG 3 1 2006		
FEB 2 5 2003			
APR 1 1 2003	MAR 3 1 2007		
	APR 1 9 2007		

11-02

facelift

AT YOUR FINGERTIPS

an
aromatherapy
massage
program for
healthy skin and
a younger face

Pierre Jean Cousin

Foreword by

Shirley Price

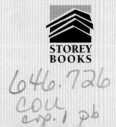

STOREY
BOOKS

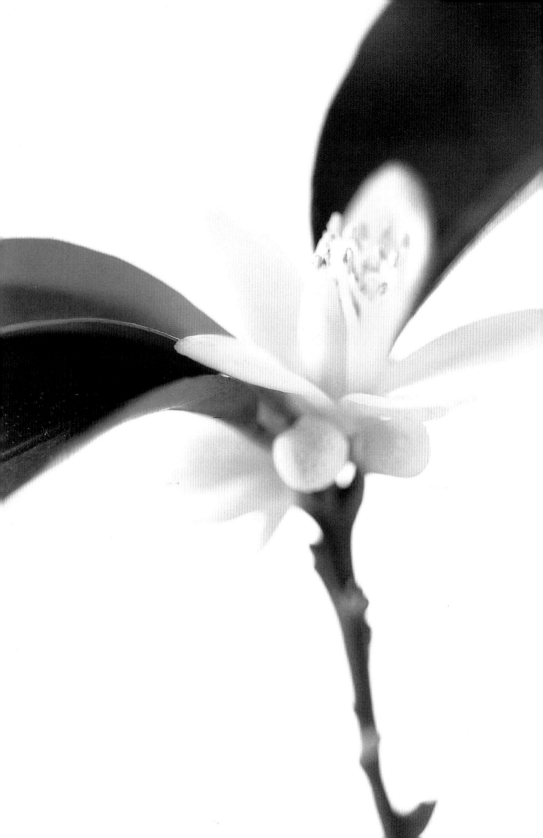

contents

foreword

Every woman wants to retain her youthful face and figure for as long as possible, but although many books have been written—and diets given—to help her keep her figure, very few have been writtten on how to preserve a youthful facial skin.

In this beautifully presented book, PJ, as he is affectionately known, has done just that—putting together a successful facial routine in which he combines the benefits of using acupressure points and therapeutic essential oils.

The healing effects of employing the pressure points of traditional Chinese medicine have been known and practiced on the body for some decades in the West, but using the same principles on the face is a fresh approach. PJ's easy-to-follow exercises and straightforward, informative text clarify and bring to the fore a subject about which not much was known or appreciated in the past.

I am delighted that in this book, which will attract many ardent followers, he emphasizes the necessity of using genuine essential oils for massage. My years of practice, experiment, and experience have taught me how greatly these can enhance results.

Follow the suggested massage program and weekly plans diligently, and you will be rewarded with a skin that will be sure to draw positive comments from your loved ones and friends.

Shirley Price
Aromatherapy Limited

introduction

Many times during my professional life as an acupuncturist and herbalist I have been asked by my clients what can be done to slow down the process of aging. We find it difficult to accept the marks of time gracefully because they affect the way we present ourselves to the world. Signs of aging can even threaten our self-esteem and self-confidence.

The conventional cosmetic approach to aging has always been fundamentally symptomatic: in focusing solely on the "problem" it ignores the person. Some single ingredient or technique is heralded as savior, and either masking or alleviating a particular symptom (such as dryness or wrinkles) is seen as the solution. The constant quest for quick-fix solutions to long-term skin problems (whether aging or some other skin condition) often fails to provide more than a very temporary camouflage of the reality, and this, in turn, inevitably generates a long succession of disappointments.

Certainly, the techniques of modern cosmetic surgery and some of the products now available may sometimes bring marked improvement, but either their benefits are so short-term or the pain, risk, and cost involved are so great that anyone with any common sense must think twice before embarking on such courses of action. General anesthetic always involves significant risk, and some of the surgical procedures available are inherently dangerous or can result in permanent scarring.

I believe that simple, natural remedies can be the basis for long-term skin care. In my practice I use a range of natural substances and techniques that are effective in the treatment of a great variety of skin conditions. Many have been used for hundreds, even thousands, of years and are, indeed, still routinely used by the cosmetics industry: essential oils and clay are among the commonest ingredients found in the lotions, creams, and masks now marketed as "natural" products.

Although natural medicine has no "cure" for aging, for what is ultimately an unstoppable, inevitable process, it can offer a better long-term approach than the regular application of expensive, relatively ineffective cosmetics or the rigors and risks of cosmetic surgery. Seen as part of a holistic approach to aging, which takes into account your general constitution as well as your present state of health, natural medicine will often trigger the spontaneous healing processes of the body while offering you the chance to become actively involved in managing your own health, beauty, and self-confidence.

My aim is to help you understand and tackle a problem that cannot be ignored or entirely resolved. The simple but effective tools I offer can improve as well as maintain your skin at little cost and without side effects. All the ingredients mentioned in the following chapters are safe to use as indicated and easily available in supermarkets, health stores, and pharmacies, or by mail order. All the techniques or procedures can be learned in a few minutes and applied immediately.

MAKING THE MOST OF THIS BOOK

The massage program (see pages 70–97) is the heart of this holistic approach to skin care: it is very important to learn all twenty steps thoroughly, so that you can perform the sequence without referring to the pictures or text. The poster is a reminder—something to pin up by your mirror or tuck into your bag as you learn.

Once you are completely familiar with the program, it should not take more than 14 minutes to complete all twenty steps twice. It is designed for long-term daily use, practiced once or twice a day for as long as possible. Start fairly intensively. The six-week programs on pages 98–103 offer useful guidance on establishing a routine and set it within the context of recipes for natural cleansing, nourishing, and toning, and a healthy diet. On page 125 there is an additional short list of acupressure points on the body—these are a valuable complement to the facial massage program.

You must assess your skin type (see page 17) and have a clear objective in mind—to detox, hydrate, tone, nourish, and so on—before you decide on your choice of oils. There are suggestions for "starter" blends of carrier and essential oils for each skin type on pages 36–37, but you need to read the sections on acupressure and aromatherapy and the oils before choosing a blend or making your own mix.

Read the section on safety precautions (pages 40–41) very carefully and take note of any contra-indications: they are important and should always be observed. If you have a common skin condition, such as acne or eczema, the index will guide you to appropriate carrier and essential oils. The oils section (pages 41–65) lists many other benefits.

Take note of the lifestyle and dietary advice on pages 13 and 122–24, too. A proper diet and vitamin or mineral supplements can make a great difference to the state of your skin.

I hope that after reading this book you will be able to make an objective assessment of your skin's condition and of how to take care of it; be able to enhance your looks and improve your self-confidence; save money usually spent on expensive cosmetic products; avoid painful, expensive treatment; and be more proactive and responsible for your appearance and your fitness. Our ability to maintain our own health or to heal ourselves is frequently underestimated or neglected. Using this book will also, I hope, help you to restore a real sense of balance in your daily life, and with that will come a more youthful face, a positive outlook, and greater well-being.

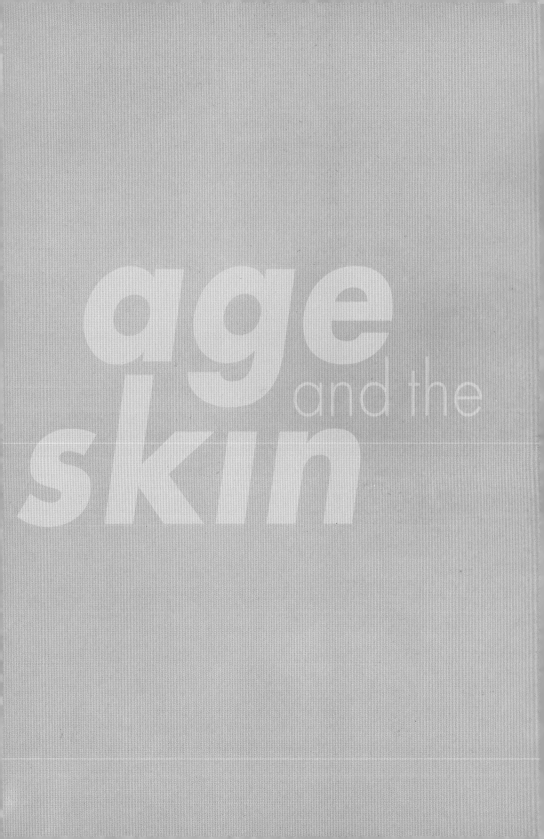

Our skin has four main functions: to protect against injuries and micro-organisms, to regulate body temperature, to receive sensations, and to eliminate toxins. Its structure is identical on every part of the body, but with important variations according to its location and function. Facial skin is adapted to monitor changes in temperature and atmospheric conditions, and also, in association with an extraordinarily complex network of muscles, to act as an important means of communication.

Examine skin under a microscope and its three different layers—epidermis, dermis, and hypodermis—are clearly apparent. The outer layer, or epidermis, made of hardwearing cells, contains no blood vessels or nerve endings. Its main functions are to protect and to regulate water evaporation. It is constantly renewed as dead cells flake off.

Below the epidermis lies the dermis. This is the most active layer of our skin—its functions are sensation, thermo-regulation, circulation, and secretion. It contains a complex structure composed of collagen, elastic fibers (called elastin), small blood vessels (or capillaries), nerve endings and the upper parts of the sebaceous and sweat glands. Collagen, a protein-based fibrous substance, plays an important part in the structure of the body. In the skin it "mingles" or associates with elastin to create "tone" or elasticity. Sebaceous glands are found almost everywhere on our bodies, except the soles of the feet and the palms of the hands. They are particularly numerous in the scalp and around the forehead, mouth, and nose, and their main function is to produce sebum, a lubricant for skin and hair. It is the changes in the dermis that are responsible for much of the aging process in skin.

The hypodermis is a layer of fatty connective tissues in which the hair follicles, as well as the base of the sebaceous and sweat glands, are located. It has a high water content.

The process of aging

Aging is a natural, slow, irreversible process of evolution which cannot be stopped. The changes that you see taking place in your face as you age are affected by subtle alterations to its anatomical structure as well as by modifications in the skin itself.

Deterioration of the skin caused by the passing of time manifests itself initially in a reduction of the life span of cells. In childhood a skin cell lives on average 100 days; for an adult, that figure is down to just 48 days. After the age of forty-five, the epidermis becomes thinner. The elastin in the dermis begins to disappear, disrupting the structure of the collagen; as a consequence, the junction between the dermis and epidermis flattens. The hypodermis is also altered as its water content diminishes—aging does dry the skin—and the distribution of its fatty cells becomes more and more uneven. All these factors contribute to an increasing lack of tone or elasticity in the skin. Later still, the fatty cells in the hypodermis begin to migrate downward, according to the law of gravity.

As your skin is subjected to structural changes it slowly becomes less efficient. Wounds take longer to heal, you bruise more easily, waste products are eliminated more slowly, your sensitivity is reduced, and blood circulation is also affected. Eventually your skin becomes more open to infections and, finally, the production of vitamin D, as well as protection against the sun, is impaired.

WRINKLES

The most obvious, enduring sign of aging in the skin is the appearance of wrinkles. They are of two different types. Expression wrinkles are mostly transverse lines, situated on the forehead, temples, and around the eyes and mouth; lowering wrinkles are mostly vertical and are caused by the changes taking place in the hypodermis.

At the age of twenty to twenty-five, small, thin wrinkles of expression appear between the eyebrows and at the outer corners of the eyes. Wrinkles around the eyes, the so-called "crow's-feet" wrinkles, are accentuated by laughing. Although not usually deep, they will be clearly defined by the age of forty.

Between twenty-five and thirty-five, transverse superficial expression wrinkles become visible on the forehead. Other small lines may appear around the mouth and vertically—these are lowering wrinkles—between the corners of the mouth and the outer sides of the nostrils. There is a slight slackening of the skin of the neck.

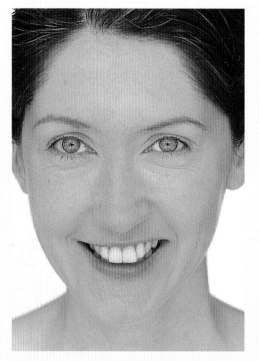 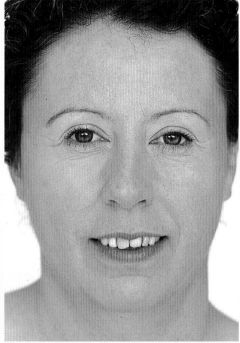

Mid thirties On this relatively young, normal skin the effects of aging are hardly visible when the face is in repose. The horizontal lines of expression are the inevitable result of a mobile face. Vertical lines of lowering have also begun to appear.

Mid forties Here the visible signs of aging are still very slight and are likely to progress slowly. This is an excellent demonstration of the one very real benefit of oily skin. The high levels of natural sebum prevent excessive and aging dehydration.

By the age of forty-five, all these wrinkles have deepened and the contour of the face is beginning to alter as the bones thin and elasticity in the skin is lost. Forty-five also marks the beginning of a definite acceleration in the natural process of aging.

Between fifty-five and sixty-five, the face begins to change its shape as the lowering of fatty tissues toward the chin and lower jaw is accelerated. The texture of the skin on the face and neck also thickens.

MAJOR ENEMIES OF THE SKIN

To a large extent the timing of the appearance of wrinkles is determined by the genetic code you inherit from your biological parents. But scientists have proved that the slow process of aging in the dermis can

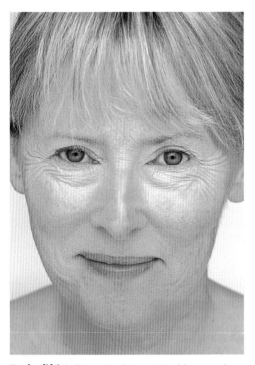

Early fifties Expression lines, vertical lines, and gradual changes in the shape of the lower part of the face are all evident. Frequent exposure to the sun can cause of loss of tone and elasticity in this type of northern, sensitive, translucent skin.

be accelerated considerably by prolonged overexposure to sunlight, smoking, and dietary imbalances. Stress can also speed the process.

The worst enemy of your skin is the sun. Only 10 percent of the sun's medium-range ultraviolet (UVB) rays penetrate through to the dermis—most get no farther than the epidermis—but it is they that act upon the all-important elastin, causing the disruption of the complex structure of collagen and the deterioration of the fibers so important to skin tone. Of course, some exposure to sunlight is essential to our well-being. It stimulates the production of vitamin D, a substance essential for the formation and maintenance of healthy bones, but regular, prolonged sunbathing is terribly destructive to the skin.

A word about sun protection products: to be on the safe side, always reduce by half the stated protection level. A cream labeled SPF 10 may offer only SPF 5 protection to anyone particularly sensitive to sunlight or to any skin type in particular conditions and situations. The effects of wind and saltwater are just two of the ways in which a factor level can be drastically altered.

Smoking is almost as great an enemy of the skin. Recent research shows that the skin of regular smokers invariably ages far more quickly than that of nonsmokers. The deterioration of elastic fibers and collagen is accelerated, and nicotine, by contracting the capillary vessels, reduces the supply of vital oxygen and nutrients to the dermis, with the inevitable consequence—the lifeless appearance of a smoker's skin.

The effects of stress on the face are well known, though they are not yet scientifically evaluated. Stress causes tension in the muscles and skin of the face. This inevitably affects the efficient functioning of the skin and accelerates the aging process. Expression wrinkles, particularly the frown lines, can be greatly accentuated as a consequence. For the negative effects of an unbalanced diet, see pages 122–24.

cosmetic solutions

The cosmetic industry's solution to the problem of aging skin has always been to offer a variety of creams and lotions. Seductively marketed with enormous reliance on poetic symbolism, they often promise a scientific miracle. In reality, the majority use two simple principles—"water in oil" or "oil in water"—to create two kinds of emulsion.

The second, oil droplets dispersed in water, is the cosmetic industry's favorite. It creates a beautifully textured cream, easy to apply and composed sometimes of up to 95 percent water. Once applied, all that expensive water evaporates without any moisturizing effect—splashing tap water on your face produces almost the same result. Such preparations were known years ago all too accurately as "vanishing creams." The other kind of emulsion—droplets of water in an oily base—has an excellent moisturizing effect. But it works not because it adds water to the skin but rather because it prevents excessive evaporation.

The liposome creams now available are no different—all follow the water-in-oil or oil-in-water formula. But, because liposomes are a phospholipid—a substance found in the cell membrane of living skin— these creams are said to penetrate the skin better and stay there longer.

SURGERY

A variety of surgical procedures are available to help give a youthful appearance to aging skin. They divide very simply into two main categories: treatment by addition (injecting collagen or silicone, or implanting gold thread) and treatment by subtraction (exfoliation, laser, or facelift). All have considerable disadvantages.

Collagen injection This involves the injection of collagen, extracted from beef cattle, along deep wrinkles to fill them up. The treatment is repeated at least once, four or five weeks later, and generally produces a very good effect. The disadvantages of collagen injections are: short-term discomfort, the risk of serious allergic reactions, and even severe disruption of the autoimmune system, the cost, and the relatively short-lived benefit. After three months, no trace of the collagen remains, but the effect will persist for at least another three months. In the most effective cases, the benefits can last as long as ten months.

A mixture of collagen and a cement used in bone surgery can also be injected to fill up deep creases. The side effects and risks are the same as for pure collagen; the results are similar, but may last for up to five years. However, mistakes cannot be corrected.

Silicone injection As with collagen, the silicone is injected straight into the tissue along deep wrinkles, but here the effect is longer lasting. However, the resulting inflammation and consequences for the autoimmune system are so severe—including weight loss, fatigue, fever, and painful joints—that this technique is illegal in many countries.

Gold-thread implantation Fine gold thread (or a material often used for ligatures in abdominal surgery) is implanted along the deeper wrinkles to fill them up. This is an expensive and painful procedure and sometimes the gold thread comes out slowly.

Exfoliation or peeling Chemical peeling removes the epidermis, and with it all the superficial wrinkles and blemishes that multiply with aging. Most commonly, an abrasive paste made from a ground stone called resorcinol is applied to the face and left for 25 minutes—three applications are necessary at 24-hour intervals. The treatment involves seven to ten days of pain (later discomfort) and confinement. For the next few months, a very strong sun screen is essential, as even mild exposure to sunlight results in some surprising pigmentation.

Another method involves the superficial burning of the skin with phenol or, more recently, with trichloroacetic acid. This expensive process is so painful that a local or even general anesthetic is necessary, and the risk of long-term scarring is high. It is now illegal in many countries.

A third exfoliation method, so-called soft peeling, uses fruit acids at varying concentration. This does not work well on damaged skin. Several treatments are needed for what is often a disappointing result, lasting a year at most. The discomfort is comparable to fairly severe sunburn.

Laser Like exfoliation, laser treatment involves the destruction of the epidermis—in this case by burning. The lasers used are not very different from surgical lasers, and treatment must therefore be carried out by a doctor: the very weak "cold" lasers used in beauty salons cannot do the job. The pain is considerable, the face will be red and covered with crust for ten days, gradually turning pink for another three or four months before a more or less normal color is re-established (irregular pigmentation is a risk). During this period, exposure to the sun may also cause erratic pigmentation. The good news is that the results of this expensive procedure (successful or otherwise) last about five years.

Facelift Cuts are made along the hairline and the skin on the face and neck is stretched upward, trimmed, and stitched into place. This is the most expensive solution. The effect is likely to last for six to ten years, and, although generally good, depends inevitably on the skill of the surgeon. It entails all the risks associated with a general anesthetic and heavy surgical intervention. Repeat treatment tends to create the bony, immobile appearance of a mummy.

types of skin

There are five basic skin types. Before embarking on the massage program, you need to be sure which type you are. To find out, use the simple test opposite. Skin condition can change over time and according to your health, so do it even if you think you are sure of the result.

Normal skin This is the ideal skin type—firm, supple, neither dry nor greasy, without spots or blemishes, and warm to the touch. Pale skins will be pink in color.

Dry skin Often slightly hot to the touch, dry skin has a tendency to powdery scaling. It is prone to early, very fine, expression wrinkles and frequently has a dull appearance. Pale skins will normally be pink but a regular smoker may look gray. Dry skin is very sensitive to cold and wind, to central heating or air conditioning, and is in constant need of moisturizer.

Oily skin Shiny, frequently with pimples and small inflamed areas, prone to acne and dermatitis, oily skin is difficult to clean, as the over-production of sebum (see page 10) gives it an unkempt look only half an hour after using a cleanser. This type of skin responds adversely to alcohol, poor diet, stress, and cold, damp winters. The good news is that oily skin tends to age more slowly because sebum naturally pre-vents water loss.

Combination skin A dry skin with shiny, oily areas (usually on the fore-head, sides of the nose, and around the mouth and chin), combination skin is difficult to maintain because parts of the face need deep mois-turizing while other areas demand astringent, drying treatment.

Aging skin Also known as mature skin, this type tends toward dryness, lacks tone, and may also be blemished or damaged, and hot or flushed with erythema (see page 19). Aging skin needs lots of attention, with the constant use of toner, hydrating lotions, and nourishing masks.

You will encounter the term "damaged skin" throughout this book. Damage is clearly a relative term. Anyone who has suffered from the more serious skin problems listed on pages 18–19 is likely to have areas of dam-aged skin. But equally all of us, especially as we grow older, will have small blemishes—areas of irregular pigmentation or scars, for example.

ASSESSING YOUR SKIN TYPE

Clean your face with warm water using cotton balls. Dry lightly with a soft towel and leave for about 30 minutes. Carefully separate one layer (or ply) from a family-size paper tissue and cover your face with it. Press lightly all over. After about a minute remove gently and exam-ine the tissue near a light or window.

Oily stains over most of paper: your skin type is oily.

Oily patches at sides of nose, around mouth and forehead: you have combination skin.

Faint oily traces over most of paper: you have normal skin.

No oily traces: your skin type is dry—often the case for mature skin.

common skin problems

Below is a glossary of common skin conditions. Essential oils, which are antibacterial, anti-inflammatory, hydrating, and regenerating, and are able to regulate the production of sebum, constitute the best alternative to conventional treatments with their long-term side effects. Recommendations are listed in the oils section (see pages 48–65).

Acne This condition is caused by a hereditary sensitivity of the sebaceous glands (see page 10) to even tiny amounts of testosterone, a male hormone secreted in varying amounts by both males and females. Diet, stress, and sunlight can affect acne for better or for worse. It is important to keep the skin clean, but resist the temptation to squeeze the small fatty lumps characteristic of the condition, as this causes further inflammation and scarring. Antibiotics can prevent the proliferation of the germs that tend to multiply in the lumps. Vitamin A acid (or retinoic acid) taken internally is quite successful in removing all the symptoms of acne, but it must be used under medical supervision and only in severe cases—it is not recommended for pregnant women or for anyone wishing to become pregnant in the next few months. The treatment can have serious side effects, including arthritis and high cholesterol, and initially makes the condition much worse.

Blackheads These are classed with whiteheads and pimples. All three are, to varying degrees, the result of the condition that causes acne, that is excessive secretion of the sebaceous glands, exacerbated by localized bacterial activity.

Dermatitis A generic name for any inflammation of the skin, dermatitis can be caused by an allergic reaction, microorganisms of viral, bacterial, or fungal origin, exposure to adverse weather conditions, or inflamed sweat glands. It may be either a temporary or a chronic condition, and it is often painful. Conventional medicine recommends an antibiotic/steroid approach, whose benefits disappear when the treatment ends.

Eczema The symptoms are a rash characterized by scaling of the skin, itching, swelling, and blistering. It can affect the face and any part of the body. For conventional treatment, see *Dermatitis*.

Ephelis See *Freckles*.

Erythema This hereditary condition, found more frequently in women, is a redness of the skin due to the dilation of small capillaries in the dermis. For conventional treatment, see *Laser* on page 16.

Freckles Very small areas of pigmentation, freckles are usually found in abundance on the face, arms, and legs in fair-skinned or red-haired people. When exposed to the sun, the pigmented areas join together to form larger patches. For conventional treatments, see *Exfoliation* and *Laser* on pages 15 and 16.

Pimples See *Blackheads*.

Psoriasis In this hereditary condition excessive numbers of cells accumulate in the epidermis, causing inflammation and flaking. Although psoriasis is technically incurable, sufferers often experience long-term remission. Sunlight is very effective in improving a psoriatic skin; olive oil blended with bergamot (an essential oil containing psoralen, a molecule which makes the skin more sensitive to UVB rays, see page 13) is also recommended and is without major side effects.

Rosacea This inflammation of the skin is characterized by a multitude of extremely small red spots on and around the nose and cheeks. The symptoms appear suddenly, with a burning or itching sensation, and may subside for a while and then reappear equally violently; at a later stage of chronic rosacea, congestion and deformation of the affected area (and particularly the nose) may require cosmetic surgery. In the earlier stages vitamin A acid can be effective (see *Acne*), but only under medical supervision.

Seborrheic dermatitis Caused by hyperactive sebaceous glands, this inflammation—in which yeast organisms are always present—affects mainly people with oily or combination skins. The forehead and sides of the nose are initially affected; then inflammation spreads rapidly to the rest of the face, which begins to look sunburned. At this later stage there is often a rather unpleasant burning sensation. The condition responds to fungicidal preparations and is made considerably worse by the application of steroid and cortisone creams.

Whiteheads See *Blackheads*.

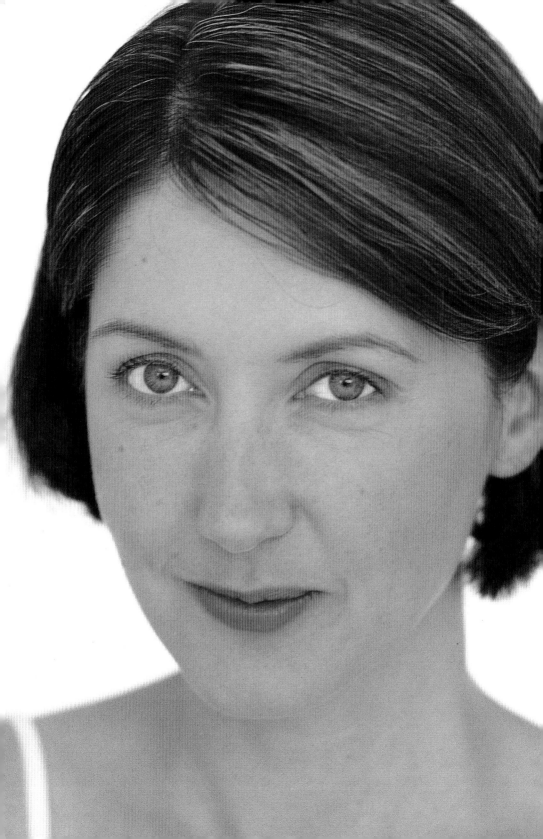

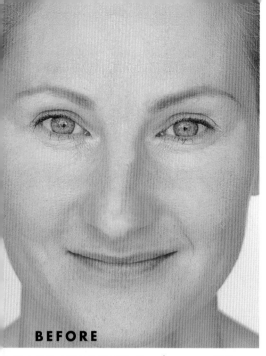

BEFORE

Sandra (normal/dry skin) noticed a definite improvement.

"The lines around my eyes and between my eyebrows have softened, and my skin tone has improved. I find it very relaxing, particularly at the end of a hard day."

CASE HISTORY: Sandra, age **39**

Acupressure and aromatherapy have been used for thousands of years for beauty and health. Bringing them together in this massage program reinforces the inherent benefit of each method but also forces them to act in synergy, producing a result greater than the sum of their individual effects.

Initially, the benefit of acupressure massage is to some extent mechanical. Rubbing and pressure simply stimulate the circulation of blood and fluids, benefiting the muscle tone and the functions of both the dermis and hypodermis (see page 10). But the stimulation of the acupressure points also triggers a natural healing process, which, in conjunction with essential oils, reduces inflammation and destroys undesirable micro-organisms. The end result is to clear the skin more effectively than any ordinary cosmetic treatment and at about one-tenth the cost.

Regular use of acupressure massage with essential oils initiates a more profound form of healing. The energizing effect achieved by stimulating acupressure points is reinforced by the regenerative, regulating properties of the essential oils so that the skin is revitalized, toxins are eliminated more effectively, fluids and temperature are regulated, and the toning of the underlying facial muscles begins. Fatty deposits along

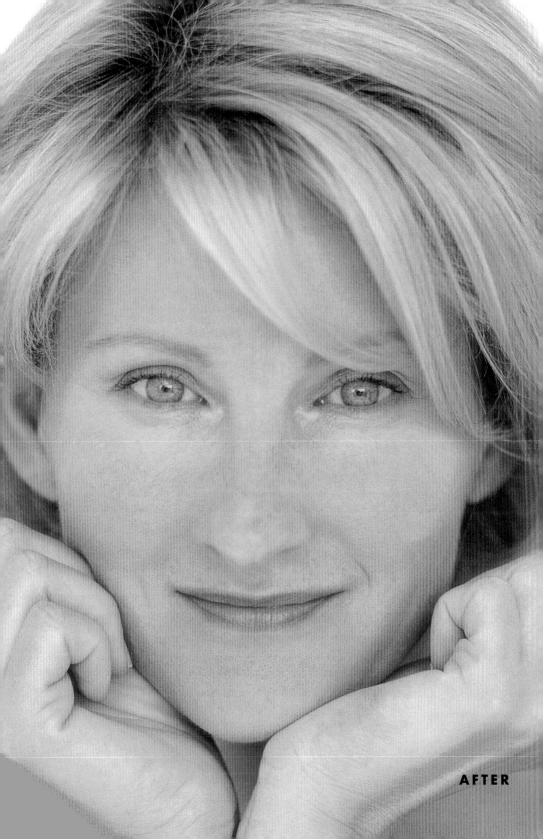

AFTER

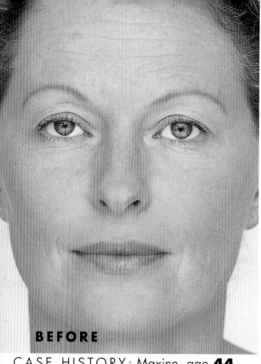

BEFORE

CASE HISTORY: Maxine, age **44**

Maxine (lucky possessor of a normal skin) is a total convert.

"I really enjoy the process. It's a simple technique that improved my appearance very quickly. Wrinkles and lines have become less apparent, my skin texture and tone are better, and its color is lighter and more even."

the jawline may gradually disappear and fine lines may fill up. But, most important of all, by using the program reasonably regularly, you can in time slow down the loss of elastin and the breakup of collagen—the main causes of wrinkling (see page 11). In addition, at this stage judicious application of the appropriate essential oils can help heal scars, repair tissue, hydrate the skin, and regulate sebum.

Results are difficult to predict because so much is dependent upon the condition of your skin when you begin, but the following indications are realistic if you establish a regular routine.

Late twenties and early thirties After five or six weeks, there will be visible changes in the tone and color of the skin. Continue with the program to maintain a healthy, youthful skin.

Late thirties and early forties After six weeks or more, fine wrinkles may fade, and there should be a definite improvement in the color, tone, and general appearance of the skin. You may also begin to see some firming on the jawline.

Late forties onward After eight to ten weeks, the quality of the skin should be much improved, and the jawline should be firmer. It is important to continue the massage program to consolidate progress.

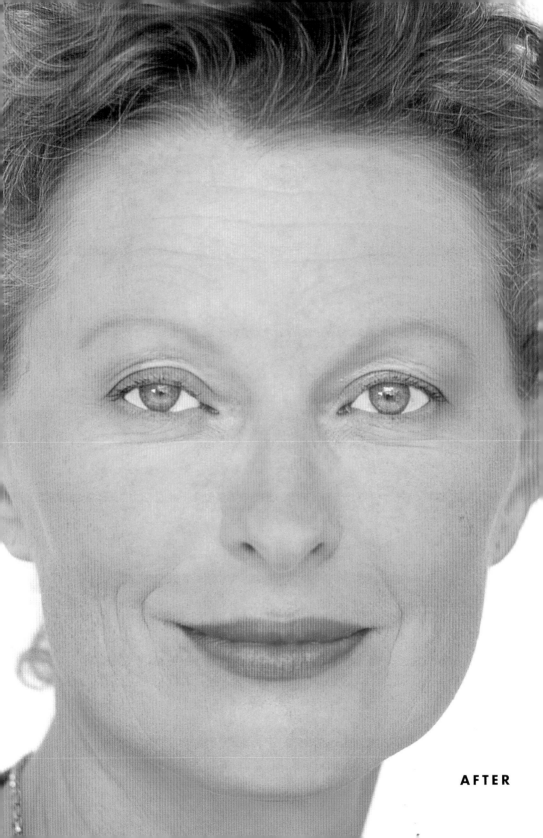

AFTER

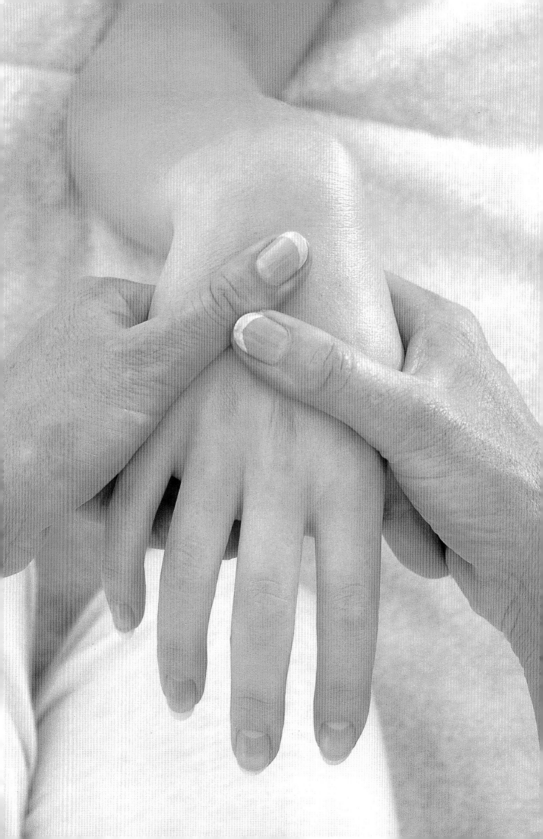

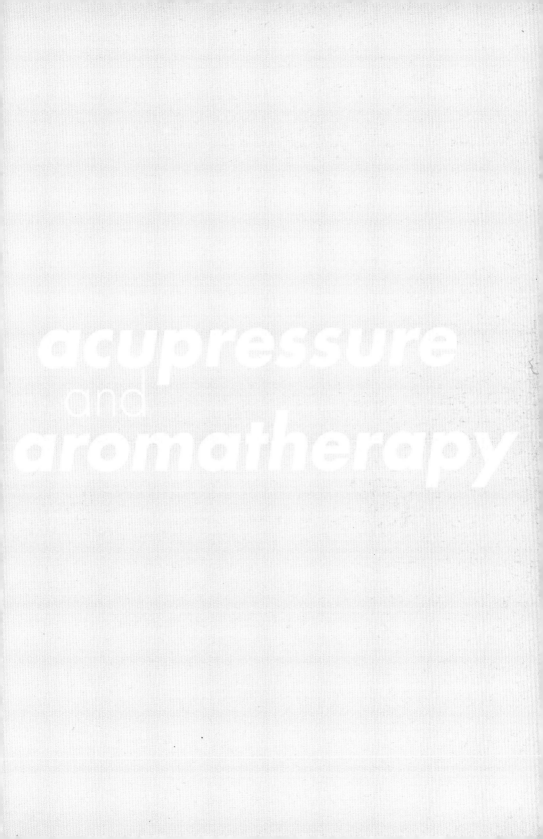

acupressure
and
aromatherapy

The massage program in this book (see pages 70–97) uses a potent new combination of acupressure and aromatherapy. In essence, the acupressure technique stimulates points on the face to activate the body's healing processes, release toxins, stimulate the circulation of blood and fluids, regulate temperature, and revitalize the skin, while the essential oils (aromatherapy) help to reduce inflammation, eliminate bacteria, regulate the natural production of sebum, and regenerate the skin. This section explains the ancient principles behind those statements.

acupressure

Acupressure is part of a complex system of diagnosis and treatment called traditional Chinese medicine (or TCM) that has been practiced for thousands of years. The first book on TCM is about 2,500 years old, and archaeologists have found indications that a crude form of TCM was already in use 4,000 years ago.

Today, TCM is widely used in China, Japan, Vietnam, Korea, and, indeed, throughout Asia. Acupressure remains a simple method of self help among oriental women, devised to maintain a youthful appearance for as long as possible. They usually practice the technique daily, using herbal creams or ointments, and back them up by taking herbal potions for enhanced vitality.

To understand exactly how acupressure works and why it can be used to rejuvenate the face and heal skin problems according to the principles of TCM is a vast and interesting subject totally outside the scope of this book. However, there are two fundamental concepts that must be explained if you are to put the techniques of the massage program into context.

UNDERSTANDING YIN AND YANG

The concept of yin and yang forms the cornerstone of TCM. There is a variety of interpretations for the meaning of the terms, but literal translation of the characters suggests "the shady side of the hill" for yin and "the sunny side of the hill" for yang. Yin characteristics are said to be darkness, cold, stillness, and heaviness; yang is said to relate more to light, heat, movement, volatility, and fire. By extension yin is perceived as a more static, solid state, while yang is a predominantly dynamic, more immaterial and inconsistent state.

Every object and every person on earth exists in a dynamic, ever-changing balance between yin and yang. Each state depends upon the other for definition—they are, in other words, aspects of the same phenomenon. One cannot exist without the other. Take the example of day changing into night: yang reaches its peak at midday, and from that moment yang swings toward yin until it reaches its peak at midnight, when it begins the swing back to yang and midday. The same is true of the year, with yang dominant in summer, yin in winter.

Since TCM states that where there is balance there is health, disease is seen as the consequence of an imbalance between yin and yang. When one becomes dominant, it has a tendency to weaken the other. An increase in heat (or yang) in the body, for example, will dry out fluids (or yin); since one of the functions of body fluid is to cool the body, an excess of heat creates a deficiency of coolness. To act on the relationship between yin and yang is the main objective of TCM, and this is achieved by working upon the blood, upon other bodily fluids and, most importantly of all, upon the Qi.

UNDERSTANDING QI OR VITAL ENERGY

Qi (pronounced chi) is the vitality or energy inherent in every human being. On the surface of the skin, Qi manifests itself in the luminosity or "shine" you see on a healthy person's face. If the level, quality, or flow of a person's Qi is poor, illness occurs; death could be defined as the total absence of Qi. Qi has a dynamic, yet synthetic, relationship with the fluids in the body. Fluids, to a certain extent, nourish Qi and influence its yin/yang balance. Yet Qi "energizes" water and circulates blood, which without Qi is an inert substance.

Qi is given different names according to the different functions it performs, among them: constitutional Qi (Yuan), nutritive Qi (Ying Qi), and the more superficial, defensive Qi (Wei Qi). Every type of Qi plays a role in transforming the human body, from conception through all the stages of life, transporting nutrients, maintaining organs in their places, enabling the body to stand erect, protecting it from disease, and maintaining a constant temperature.

Qi is carried through the body in a series of channels or pathways called jing-luo. The word is commonly translated as meridian, from "jing" ("to go through" or "a thread in a fabric") and "luo" ("something that connects or attaches" or "a net"). Meridians carry blood as well as Qi, but they are not blood vessels. Rather, they consist of an invisible network that links together every part of the body, internally and externally. Although the meridian system is unseen, it is thought to embody a physical reality essential for maintaining the harmonious balance of yin and yang.

There are twelve main meridians running bilaterally and longitudinally on the surface of the body, but connecting at a deeper level to all the vital organs, so enabling an even distribution of blood and Qi to every part of the body. These channels are named after the organ they affect most—for example, the heart, small intestine, stomach, and liver meridians—and each is classified yin or yang, acccording to that organ's energy within the body.

When Qi gets blocked, stagnates, or does not flow well, the yin/yang balance is profoundly disturbed, and illness—physical, mental, or emotional—occurs. Acupressure massage is one of the four ways in which TCM treats disorders of Qi (the others are acupuncture, changes in diet, and herbal treatments). By massaging specific points of the meridian system, acupressure is designed to free and direct the flow of Qi within the body, as well as to improve its level and quality. A less extreme, less invasive form of treatment than acupuncture, it is slower to take effect, but its action upon the skin and general health can ultimately be more comprehensive.

aromatherapy

Aromatic essential oils were first distilled in Ancient Egypt c. 3000 B.C., and they have been used ever since in massage, in the bath, and for cosmetic purposes in scenting the hair and the body. By Ancient Greek and Roman times, essential oils (in particular, basil, oregano, thyme, and rose) were also renowned for their therapeutic importance.

Scientific research in the twentieth century has confirmed the medicinal worth of many essential oils, demonstrating, for example, that they are capable of destroying or inhibiting viruses and bacteria, combating inflammation, or regulating hormones. It was a Frenchman, R. M. Gattefossé, who coined the word "aromatherapy" in 1928, and his research in the field of aromatic plants is the foundation of the modern approach to essential oils. Today aromatherapists use essential oils to soothe, stimulate, or heal the body, the mind, and the emotions.

EXPLAINING ESSENTIAL OILS

The oils are found in the roots, leaves, stems, or flowers of aromatic plants, in the bark of some trees (such as pine, fir, or cinnamon), or in the outer peel of some citrus fruits. Essential oils can be obtained from many plants, and each oil is a complex mixture of up to 250 chemicals. Most of these fragrant substances are extracted by the ancient process of steam distillation. A few, such as the citrus oils, are obtained by cold pressing, and others, such as jasmine, by chemical extraction; the latter are called "absolutes."

Essential oils are an excellent alternative to the skin conditioning and treatment offered by cosmetic products and conventional medicine. Provided that the safety precautions and instructions concerning blending are followed, they are perfectly safe to use at home. Their chemistry is so complex that it is impossible to know exactly how they work, although scientific classification of their molecules has helped to explain some of their therapeutic effects. The most important chemical groups found in essential oils are set out opposite. How much (if any) of these substances is found in each particular oil will determine how safe it is to use and its therapeutic value.

Monoterpenes Occurring in almost all essential oils, these substances are antiseptic, analgesic, and stimulating. Oils rich in monoterpenes—thyme is one example—can irritate the skin in large doses and should be used with caution.

Sesquiterpenes These are antiseptic, but also anti-inflammatory, calming, and analgesic. The oils rich in sesquiterpenes are non-toxic and usually well tolerated by the skin. German and Roman chamomile oils both contain sesquiterpenes. Diterpenes, part of the same chemical family, are also fungicidal and antiviral.

Alcohols Powerful anti-infective, antiviral, and bactericidal agents, the alcohols are stimulating to the skin, although their action upon it is gentle and non toxic. Lavender, tea tree, geranium, and clary sage oils all contain important aromatic alcohols.

Phenols Another antiseptic group, the phenols stimulate the central nervous system and activate the body's own healing process. However, due to their potential toxicity and their aggressive action on the skin, oils rich in phenols, such as red thyme and cinnamon, should be left to qualified aromatherapists.

Aldehydes Substances in this group are antiviral, anti-inflammatory, antipyretic (effective against fever), and calming to the nervous system.

Ketones Analgesic, anti-inflammatory, cicatricial (effective in helping to build new tissue), and sedative, these substances are toxic and must be avoided if pregnant. Some types of rosemary oil are rich in ketones.

Esters Fungicidal, anti-inflammatory, antispasmodic, and cicatricial, esters are also beneficial to the nervous system. Roman chamomile oil contains up to 75–80 percent esters.

Oxides These substances are expectorant but can be irritating to the skin. Oil containing oxides (for example, certain types of eucalyptus) should be used with caution.

Lactones and Furocoumarins The main causes of phototoxicity—that is they will make the skin change color when exposed to strong sunlight—these substances are also antipyretic. Some types of citrus fruit oil, such as mandarin, are rich in both.

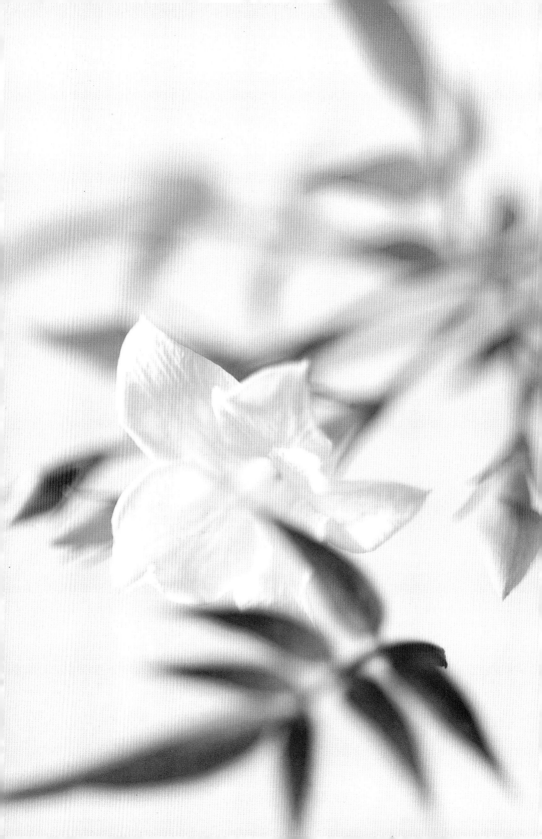

choosing your oils

If you are eager to get started and have never used essential oils in massage before, the choices before you can seem bewildering. But the tables of carrier and essential oils on pages 66–69 can help you organize your options, and so can the suggestions and recommendations set out below. Just remember: these are designed simply as a starting point for your own experiments, based on the detailed information given in this section. You alone can assess what your skin type is—if you haven't done the tissue test yet, do it now (see page 17).

normal skin

OBJECTIVE   To maintain and nourish

CARRIER OIL   1 tbsp. sweet almond *or* olive

ESSENTIAL OIL   Choose any **three** from the following, using three drops of each: geranium, lavender, jasmine, neroli, rose otto, rosewood, and sandalwood

RECOMMENDED BLENDS
1. lavender and rosewood to cleanse; geranium to hydrate
2. rose otto and neroli to hydrate and tone; sandalwood to balance natural sebum

dry skin

OBJECTIVE   To cool and hydrate

CARRIER OIL   1 tbsp. apricot kernel *or* lime blossom *or* olive *or* ¾ tbsp. of **one** of the above plus ¼ tsp. wheatgerm *or* borage

ESSENTIAL OIL   Choose any **three** from the following, using three drops of each: clary sage, frankincense, geranium, lavender, Roman chamomile, rose otto, sandalwood

RECOMMENDED BLENDS
1. geranium to hydrate; Roman chamomile to cool; sandalwood to balance natural sebum
2. Roman chamomile to cool; clary sage to hydrate; frankincense to repair and prevent wrinkles

oily skin

OBJECTIVE	To clean and close pores
CARRIER OIL	1 tbsp. hazelnut *or* olive *or* calendula *or* ¾ tbsp. of **one** of the above plus ¼ tsp. jojoba *or* macadamia nut
ESSENTIAL OIL	Choose **two** from the following, using five drops of each: cedarwood, chamomile (either type), geranium, lavender, mandarin, myrrh, niaouli, palmarosa, patchouli, rosewood

RECOMMENDED BLENDS
1. cedarwood to regulate pores; chamomile for inflammation
2. geranium to hydrate; lavender to cleanse, regulate, and calm irritation

combination skin

OBJECTIVE	To clean and hydrate
CARRIER OIL	1 tbsp. hazelnut *or* hypericum *or* olive *or* lime blossom
ESSENTIAL OIL	Choose any **three** from the following, using three drops of each: cedarwood, chamomile (either type), cypress, geranium, lavender, myrrh, palmarosa, rose otto, sandalwood, tea tree

RECOMMENDED BLENDS
1. cedarwood to regulate; chamomile to calm irritation; geranium to hydrate
2. lavender to calm irritation; myrrh to repair; sandalwood to tone and balance

aging skin

OBJECTIVE	To hydrate, nourish, and tone
CARRIER OIL	1 tbsp. avocado *or* apricot kernel *or* lime blossom *or* olive *or* ¾ tbsp. of **one** of the above plus ¼ tsp. wheatgerm *or* borage *or* macadamia nut
ESSENTIAL OIL	Choose any **two** from the following, using five drops of each: clary sage, cypress, frankincense, geranium, lavender, neroli, palmarosa, rose otto, sandalwood

RECOMMENDED BLENDS
1. clary sage to hydrate and regulate; neroli to tone
2. palmarosa to regenerate; rose otto to hydrate and tone

CHOOSING YOUR CARRIER

Before you can start blending your chosen essential oils, you need to select a single carrier oil or a carrier mixture. Carrier oils are the vegetable oils needed to dilute the essential oils used for massage. In theory, any vegetable oil would do; in reality, cold-pressed oils obtained from nuts or seeds have specific therapeutic properties and often act in synergy with the essential oils selected; that is, they work together with them to produce an effect greater than the sum of the individual essential oils.

Top-quality cold-pressed carrier oils are expensive, but a small quantity goes a long way. They are also immensely more beneficial to the skin than their industrially extracted counterparts, because, unlike the latter, they retain a valuable mixture of vitamins, trace elements, and fatty acids in varying quantity. Olive, sweet almond, and wheatgerm oil are easily available almost everywhere, while all the other oils can be ordered from the reputable specialists listed on page 126.

From the twelve carrier oils that are featured in this section (see pages 41–47), you will probably need to choose one, possibly two, that are suitable for your skin before adding essential oils. Carrier oils are mixed for one or more of three basic reasons—to enhance a therapeutic effect, to reduce cost, or to improve penetration. Calendula and hypericum carrier oils, for example, act in synergy and are particularly effective in the treatment of skin inflammation, oily, or damaged skin.

It is best to try one carrier at a time. First impressions are often correct—if it feels good, it is very likely to be appropriate—but do not rely on intuition alone. Make sure you have properly assessed your skin type and its condition first (see pages 8–19). The correct choice of a carrier oil is very important. It will have a profound influence on the state of your skin and will determine how quickly you are able to see positive results.

CHOOSING ESSENTIAL OILS

To your single carrier oil or the carrier mixture of your choice you may add, according to the principles of traditional Chinese medicine, up to four essential oils (see pages 48–65).

The first essential oil you choose should be selected to realize your main objective: it might be to moisturize your skin, to regulate the natural production of sebum (see page 10), or to reduce wrinkles. If you have aging (dry) skin, for example, you may decide to use geranium.

Next, you may if you wish choose one or two essential oils that will enhance or complement your first choice. Clary sage and neroli oil, for example, would both complement geranium very well by toning and hydrating aging skin.

Finally, you may choose one more essential oil, either to counteract any possible over-action of the main essential oil or to treat some other existing skin problem. Chamomile, for example, would certainly help if there were any inflammation of the skin.

For all practical purposes you will probably use only two or three essential oils. But, whether you choose to use one or four, the total quantity of essential oil should never be more than 3.5 percent of your final preparation. The viscosity of carrier and essential oils differs, and there are differences of volume between the different carriers and essential oils, too; so it is impossible to be precise about quantities without resorting to a chemistry set. However, you can work completely safely on the basis that to every ⅓ fl.oz. (10ml.) of carrier oil you can add a maximum of ten drops of essential oil. This means that if you are blending two essential oils, you can use a maximum of five drops of each, while for a blend of three you should use no more than three drops of each oil.

PREPARING YOUR MASSAGE OIL

As you are likely to be experimenting with various mixes, it is best to make only a very small amount at first. One tablespoon of carrier oil and a blend of ten drops of essential oil will be enough for two days' massage, morning and evening. Once you are satisfied with a blend, prepare a larger amount in advance; it will keep for several months. Many people use too much oil when they begin massage, but it does not take long to become accustomed to the sequences, and a massage oil preparation containing 1¾ fl.oz. (50ml.) of carrier oil(s) and 50 drops of essential oil should last you about two weeks.

You can buy glass bottles fitted with removable droppers at specialty aromatherapy shops and many pharmacies (see page 126 for mail-order sources). They are usually available in a variety of sizes; you will need at least two—a large one for assembling your preparation and a small one for blending your essential oils before adding them to the carrier. Pour the appropriate amount of carrier oil (or oils) into the larger bottle first. Next assemble your essential oils in the small bottle, adding the dropper and stopper, and shake well to blend. Then put the essential oils in the larger bottle, add the stopper, shake again, and your preparation is ready to use.

The tables on pages 66–69 provide a quick-reference overview of the carrier and essential oils described earlier in this section. Both are designed to help you compare relative values when you are making your selection. On pages 36–37 you will find suggestions for several blends for your skin type. Based on the principles set out above, they offer a simple starting point and the basis for your first experiments.

SAFETY NOTE

Most essential oils are perfectly safe for home use, provided they are used correctly. However, they are powerful substances, so some precautions must be taken. Always store the bottles out of sunlight, and never let the oils come into contact with your eyes—even diluted essential oil will make them sting. If diluted essential oil is splashed into the eyes, flush them immediately with a carrier oil or vegetable oil. If the essential oil is neat, flush immediately—ideally using milk (or with a carrier or vegetable oil)—and, if the irritation persists, seek medical assistance right away.

Although most essential oils should be diluted in a carrier oil before use, lavender can be used neat on a burn; undiluted tea tree oil can treat athlete's foot; and jasmine, rose attar, or sandalwood can be used directly on the skin as a perfume. Juniper oil should always be used with care, as it can sometimes cause a mild skin irritation. When using a citrus oil, such as mandarin, avoid immediate exposure to strong sunlight or the ultraviolet light of a sunbed.

As with all concentrated substances, you must keep essential oils out of the reach of children; never leave a bottle without a fixed dropper where a child could take off the cap and consume the contents. Do not, unless otherwise advised by an expert and with the few exceptions mentioned above, apply neat essential oil to the skin.

Oils in pregnancy Most essential oils are best avoided during the first months of pregnancy. After the third or fourth month, still avoid using cedarwood, clary sage, and juniper oils. However, there are many other oils that are safe to use during this time, including chamomile, geranium, jasmine, lavender, neroli, patchouli, rose attar, and sandalwood.

carrier oils

apricot kernel

A rich, nourishing oil recommended for dry skin, apricot kernel also protects and lubricates the skin, as well as calming the inflammation or irritation of dermatitis and eczema. It can also be used on normal skin or as a preventive measure against exposure to cold wind during winter vacations. It contains vitamins (A, B1, B2, B6 and E), traces of calcium, phosphorus, potassium and sulfur, and polyunsaturated, as well as monounsaturated, fatty acid.

COMBINES WELL WITH: an equal quantity of hypericum oil for a much-enhanced cooling, anti-inflammatory effect. For mature skin, the addition of 5 percent borage oil is very useful; lime blossom oil added in equal quantity will help diminish small, superficial lines.

avocado

This cloudy, sometimes even sludgy, oil is excellent for treating dry skin and wrinkles. Cold pressed from the flesh of the avocado, it contains vitamins, antioxidants, lecithin, and trace minerals. Avocado is cooling and anti-inflammatory and penetrates well into the skin. (See page 115 for an avocado facial mask—an alternative treatment if avocado oil is not available.)

COMBINES WELL WITH: approximately 85 percent of a more fluid oil, such as grapeseed or sweet almond oil.

calendula

This oil is recommended for mixed and oily skins. It is a maceration oil, made by soaking the flowers of *Calendula officinalis* in sunflower oil for three weeks and then carefully filtering the mixture, which has extraordinary healing properties. Gently cooling and slightly drying, it is used mainly for the healing of scars. Rich in carotene, saponins, and bitter principles, this oil is an excellent anti-inflammatory, fungicidal, and antibacterial agent—a must for any chronically damaged skin.

COMBINES WELL WITH: equal quantities of hazelnut or hypericum oil. For eczema, try a mix of equal parts of calendula, arnica, and hypericum oil. If the skin is very inflamed, applications of, alternately, calendula oil and aloe vera gel give excellent results.

grapeseed

A safe, neutral, and very inexpensive oil, grapeseed is an excellent carrier for any essential oil. It is of little therapeutic value on its own, except for its vitamin E content and its good skin penetration.

COMBINES WELL WITH: more powerful and expensive carriers, which makes it an excellent medium for dilution. It can be used in equal quantities as a moderator for a strongly scented carrier (such as olive oil) or an astringent (such as hazelnut oil). It is also an excellent neutral base, used alone, with a little wheatgerm oil, or with 10–20 percent borage or macadamia nut oil.

hazelnut

This carrier is particularly recommended to use on its own for oily skin because it helps to regulate sebum (the natural oily secretion of the skin). Rich in oleic and linoleic acid, it also contains trace elements of copper and iron. With its astringent properties and exceptional ability to penetrate and diffuse into the skin, it is very helpful in the treatment of acne, dermatitis, and seborrheic eczema.

COMBINES WELL WITH: either calendula (to speed skin regeneration) or hypericum (to reduce inflammation) in equal quantities, but best used alone.

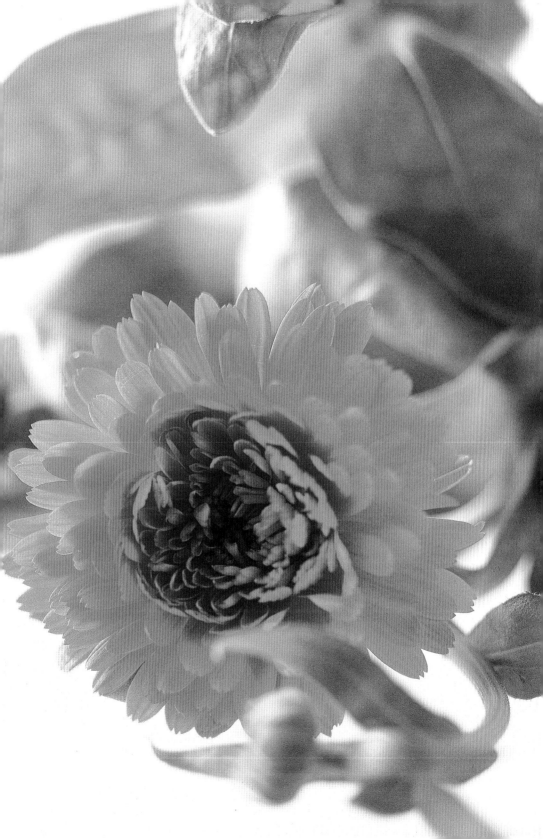

hypericum (St. John's wort)

Another maceration oil (see calendula, page 42), the St. John's wort flowers in olive oil must be exposed to strong sunlight for three weeks, during which time the active substance (called hypericin) diffuses, giving the oil a rich, deep red color. Hypericum oil is a suitable carrier for all types of skin, especially if oily and/or inflamed. It is also recommended for damaged skin, eczema, and dermatitis.

COMBINES WELL WITH: an equal quantity of calendula oil for a strong synergistic action against any inflammation.

jojoba

Extracted from the beans of a South American plant, jojoba oil contains substances similar to our sebum (see hazelnut, page 42). This thick, highly penetrative oil suits all skin types but is better diluted with other, lighter carriers. It is recommended for skin inflammation, acne, eczema, and psoriasis.

COMBINES WELL WITH: 85–90 percent of a more fluid oil, such as calendula, grapeseed, hazelnut, or sweet almond.

lime blossom (linden blossom)

The third maceration oil (see calendula, page 42), this one uses the flowers of *Tilia* x *europaea*, a tree commonly found in northern Europe. It is very good for sensitive or aging skin and is also said to have a beneficial effect on small, superficial wrinkles. Calming and gently anti-inflammatory, this delicately scented oil can be used by itself or in a variety of combinations.

COMBINES WELL WITH: 10 percent borage, jojoba, macadamia nut, or wheatgerm oil.

macadamia nut

This richly textured oil, a must for dry, aging skin, originates in Australia. One of its active ingredients is palmitoleic acid, a natural substance similar to our sebum (see hazelnut, page 42).

COMBINES WELL WITH: 80–90 percent apricot kernel, lime blossom, or sweet almond oil as a perfect carrier for a mature skin; a small amount of borage oil (approx. 5 percent) can also be added for enhanced effect.

olive

Used on the skin for centuries, olive oil is still one of the best carrier oils. It is easily available and relatively inexpensive, but be sure to use only extra virgin, cold-pressed oil. Italian olive oil is particularly good, being lighter and not too heavily scented. Olive oil is rich in oleic and linoleic acid and arachidin and palmitin—two important polyunsaturated fatty acids which help in the treatment of skin inflammations, burns and other scars, and arteriosclerosis. It is better used in diluted form with a lighter carrier.

COMBINES WELL WITH: an equal quantity of grapeseed oil. It can also be combined with equal amounts of calendula or hypericum oil for a stronger effect.

sweet almond

A favorite among aromatherapists, this oil is a versatile carrier, blending with any other oil and penetrating the skin very well. It is excellent for most types of skin and contains both oleic and linoleic acid in small amounts, vitamins A and B, minerals (copper and iron), and trace elements. Similar in many ways to apricot-kernel oil (see page 41), sweet almond is not so rich, but more easily available and cheaper.

COMBINES WELL WITH: 50 percent lime blossom oil and 5 percent borage oil for dry skin. For damaged skin, mix with an equal amount of calendula; for mature skin, mix with 10 percent borage, macadamia nut, and wheatgerm oil.

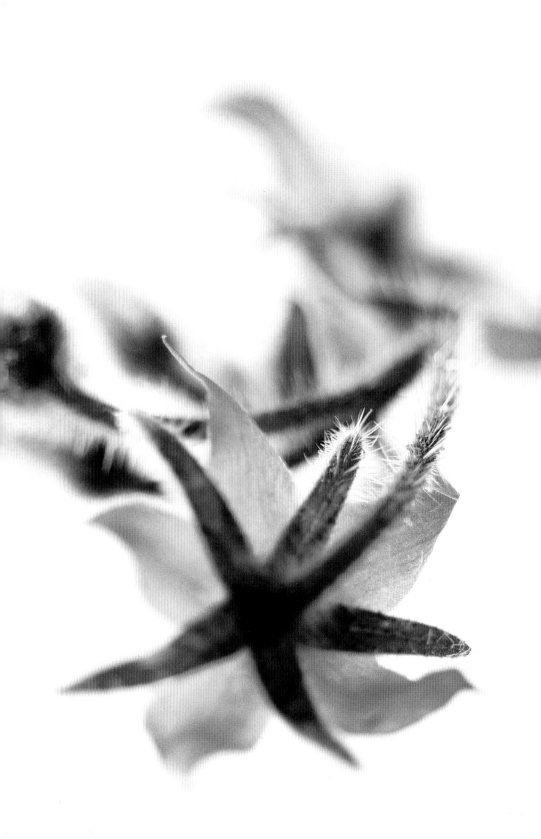

wheatgerm oil

This very sticky oil is not used on its own but is an extremely useful addition to any other carrier oil. Suitable for all skin types but particularly for dry skin, it contains protein and minerals and is high in vitamin E—all recommended in the treatment of eczema, psoriasis, and prematurely aged skin.

COMBINES WELL WITH: 80–90 percent apricot kernel, grapeseed, lime blossom, or sweet almond oil.

supplementary oils

borage

Available in capsule form in drugstores or health-food stores, this oil is extracted from *Borago officinalis*, commonly known as the starflower, found in gardens and even on wasteland. It is added in small quantity (5–10 percent) to carrier oils and is especially useful for aging skin. Considered a more potent version of evening primrose oil, it contains 15 percent gamma linoleic acid, can play an important role in the regulation of prostaglandin, and is very helpful for dry, scaly eczema. If borage is not available, use evening primrose oil instead.

vitamin e

Essential for the healing of scars and for damaged skin, vitamin E capsules are available in most health-food stores and drugstores. Empty the contents of a few capsules to add approx. 5 percent vitamin E to the carrier oil(s) of your choice. There is no need to add extra vitamin E if you are using wheatgerm oil.

essential oils

cedarwood

Extracted from the wood of the cedar tree, this healing, regenerative oil is recommended for use on mature and damaged skin and works by stimulating the lymphatic system. However, it must be used carefully (see suitability, below) and only sparingly, as it is slightly toxic to the nervous system.

In Chinese medicine, cedarwood is regarded as slightly yin and astringent. It aids the circulation of Qi, cools, and eliminates fluids.

GOOD FOR: damaged skin, dermatitis, eliminating fatty deposits and water, reducing spider veins (small blood vessels visible under the skin), scars.

NOT SUITABLE FOR: pregnant women, babies, or young children.

COMBINES WELL WITH: carrier oils—all listed, especially calendula for damaged skin; essential oils—most, especially chamomile and lavender.

chamomile

There are two types: Roman and German chamomile. Both contain the same compound—azulene or chamazulene, a fatty substance with excellent antibacterial properties, which makes this one of the best anti-inflammatories for any type of skin.

Roman chamomile is distilled from the common chamomile (now classified by botanists and pharmacologists as *Chamaemelum nobile,* formerly known as *Anthemis nobilis*), a traditional medicinal plant used by the Greeks and Romans for its calming and anti-inflammatory properties. It is often grown in gardens and naturally re-seeds itself on wasteland. Large quantities of flowers are distilled to obtain a small amount of relatively expensive, pungent oil. The same plant is used in infusions for intestinal problems and for its calming effect on the mind.

German chamomile is distilled from the flower of *Matricaria recutita* (or *M. chamomilla*) and contains far more chamazulene than common (Roman) chamomile. It is the high content of this precious ingredient that gives the oil its extraordinary, deep blue color. German chamomile is expensive, but such a small amount is needed for such good results that it is well worth the expense.

In Chinese medicine, chamomile is a cooling, slightly yin oil which helps to circulate Qi, reduces inflammation and fever, benefits the skin, and promotes tissue repair. Chamomile is also said to calm the mind and dissipate anger, harmonize digestion, and relieve stress-related bowel disorders such as irritable bowel syndrome (IBS).

GOOD FOR: burns, dermatitis, eczema.

OTHER USES: antibacterial, anti-spasmodic, and calming—conjunctivitis, colitis, IBS, diaper rash, neuralgia, headache, irritability, rheumatism; also as an infusion for colic and mild bowel disorders in children.

COMBINES WELL WITH: carrier oils—calendula, hypericum, lime blossom, olive. For any inflammation on oily skin or for chronic seborrheic dermatitis, blend with lavender, rosewood, and tea tree in a hazelnut and macadamia nut carrier. For dry, aging skin, combine with a base of apricot kernel, borage, jojoba and lime blossom. For one of the simplest and best preparations for most types of eczema, combine with a base of calendula and hypericum.

clary sage

One of more than 200 species of sage, *Salvia sclarea,* or clary, produces from the steam distillation of its leaves, flowers, and stems a very complex oil with more than 200 constituent ingredients. The most significant of these is the relatively small amount (1.6 percent to 7 percent) of a chemical called sclareol, whose main characteristic is to mimic estrogen. This hormone-regulating oil is of great benefit for aging skin and can also be used on dry or oily skin.

In Chinese medicine, this oil is considered slightly yang. It strengthens the Qi, dispels congestion, and regulates menstruation.

GOOD FOR: acne (often swift acting), inflamed skin, wrinkles.

OTHER USES: antidepressant; fluid-regulating; hormone-regulating—hot flashes and amenorrhea (lack of periods); hypotensive—helps to lower

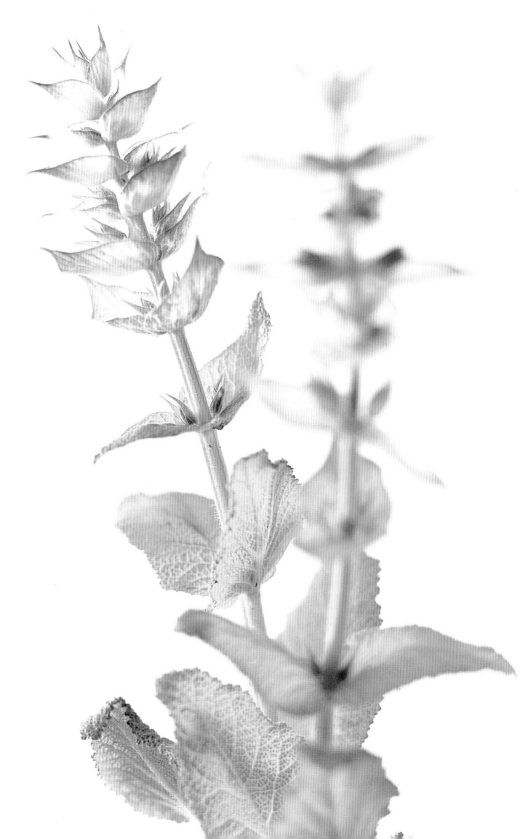

blood pressure; migraine (amazingly effective); sedative.

NOT SUITABLE FOR: pregnant women or those with a history of breast cancer; its prolonged use may also occasionally induce mild water retention.

COMBINES WELL WITH: carrier oils—apricot kernel, borage, hazelnut, hypericum, lime blossom, wheatgerm; essential oils—cedarwood, cypress, geranium, lavender, mandarin, neroli, sandalwood.

cypress

Extracted by steam distillation from the cones, flowers, twigs, and leaves of the tree, cypress oil is valued in skin care particularly for its antibacterial and astringent action on oily skin.

In Chinese medicine, this oil is considered cool, dry, astringent and slightly yin. It stimulates the reproductive form of Qi, regulates menstruation, helps the body detoxify, regulates fluid retention, and reduces inflammation.

GOOD FOR: flushed, oily skin (as in chronic erythema, rosacea, or seborrheic dermatitis), reducing spider veins.

OTHER USES: antibacterial and anti-spasmodic—eases symptoms of asthma and bronchitis; calming—extremely effective in the reduction of menopausal tension.

COMBINES WELL WITH: carrier oils—borage, calendula, hazelnut, hypericum, jojoba, macadamia nut; essential oils—chamomile, clary sage, lavender, tea tree. For antibacterial skin treatments, use a hazelnut oil base to enhance astringent properties, or a calendula and hypericum mix for a more cooling effect.

frankincense

This oil, obtained from the gum resin of the olibanum tree, has been used for thousands of years by the Egyptians, the Chinese, and the peoples of the Indian subcontinent. It is recommended as an effective, safe, anti-inflamatory and astringent for use on dry, aging skin; and these qualities and the oils immuno-stimulant properties make it a first choice to promote healing.

In Chinese medicine, this is a warm, yang oil. It encourages the circulation of blood and Qi, reduces swelling, and heals wounds.

GOOD FOR: aging neck, scars, wrinkles.

OTHER USES: astringent, anti-inflammatory, and immuno-stimulant—all effective in healing wounds.

COMBINES WELL WITH: carrier oils—apricot kernel, borage, calendula, lime blossom; essential oils—clary sage, geranium, lavender, myrrh, neroli. Combine with equal quantities of geranium and myrrh essential oils in a calendula base for an excellent mix for the neck.

geranium

Derived from *Pelargonium graveolens, P. asperum rosat,* or *P. a. bourbon*, geranium oil is one of the most useful and versatile oils for the skin. It can be used for all skin types, although its fungicidal, antibacterial, and anti-inflammatory properties are said to be most beneficial to oily skin. A complex oil containing more than 50 constituent ingredients, geranium is one of the most delicate fragrances used in perfumery and aromatherapy. Its fragrance easily dominates and "improves" the scent of oil mixes containing pungent oils such as chamomile or tea tree, but it also acts as a mosquito repellent and in summer can be included in preparations that protect the skin from sun.

In Chinese medicine, geranium is a warm, yang herb, regulating and strengthening Qi. It is considered an astringent oil with moistening properties, and is also good for fatigue and depression.

GOOD FOR: acne, burns, damaged skin, dry or weepy eczema, itchy inflamed skin, seborrheic skin, scars, wounds; also for stimulating blood circulation and constricting small blood vessels—regulating congestion, accumulated fluids, and poor elimination.

OTHER USES: regulating the endocrine system—utmost benefit for various hormone-related conditions, such as depression, fatigue, irregular or painful menstruation, premenopausal and menopausal symptoms, premenstrual syndrome (PMS), water retention.

COMBINES WELL WITH: carrier oils—all listed; essential oils—all listed.

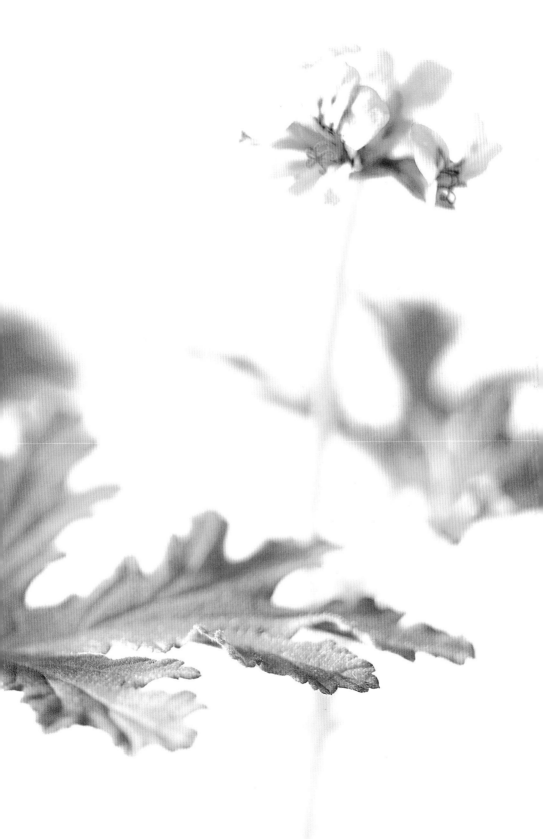

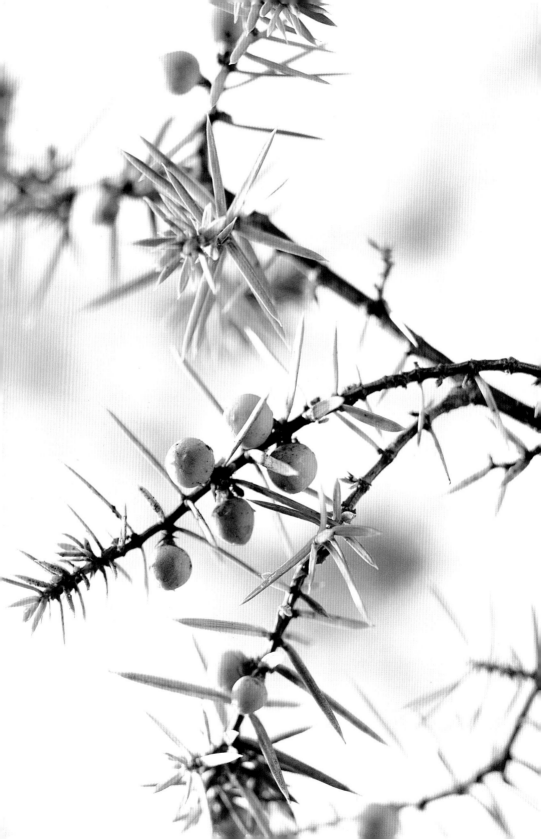

jasmine

This expensive absolute is extensively used in perfumery for its wonderful scent. A complex substance containing more than 100 constituent ingredients, it is chemically extracted from the flower and is very gentle and nontoxic. Jasmine's soothing, anti-inflammatory action is most useful for oily, mixed, and sensitive skins. Beware of cheap imitations—poor-quality jasmine is frequently adulterated and may cause adverse reactions.

In Chinese medicine, jasmine is a warm, yang oil. It stimulates the circulation of Qi, enhances yang, regulates menstruation, is often prescribed for frigidity or impotence, encourages tissue repair, alleviates pain, and moistens the skin. Jasmine is also said to alleviate labor pain and to stimulate lactation in nursing mothers.

GOOD FOR: dermatitis, pruritus (intense itching), seborrheic and sensitive skin.

OTHER USES: analgesic and anti-spasmodic—muscular pains; gently uplifting—good for depression, anxiety, and stress-related disorders; irregular menstrual periods.

COMBINES WELL WITH: carrier oils—calendula, hazelnut, jojoba, macadamia nut, olive; essential oils—chamomile, cypress, mandarin, neroli, sandalwood.

juniper

Extracted by distillation from the berries, needles, and twigs of *Juniperus communis*, this oil—always used sparingly—expels uric acid from the body and is a powerful detoxifying agent. In skin care, its antibacterial, anti-inflammatory, and healing properties are also beneficial. Juniper can be used for all skin types. The essential oil made just from juniper berries is much more expensive and is usually labeled juniper berry oil.

In Chinese medicine, juniper oil is warm, dry, and yang. It is used in winter for rheumatism and muscular pain caused by cold; it is also prescribed for a yin person with cold skin and chronic skin problems that appear to worsen in winter.

GOOD FOR: psoriasis, stretch marks, and weeping and infected eczema.

OTHER USES: anti-inflammatory—alleviating anxiety and stress; arthritis, rheumatism and stiff joints; stimulating poor circulation.

NOT SUITABLE FOR: pregnant women or for people with kidney disease.

COMBINES WELL WITH: carrier oils—calendula, hazelnut, hypericum; essential oils—clary sage, geranium, lavender, palmarosa.

lavender

A classic, sweet essence with a wonderfully evocative, Mediterranean fragrance, the lavender oil derived from the flowering tops of *Lavandula angustifolia* is probably the essential oil most frequently used by specialists, owing to its healing power and its safety. This is a good, all-purpose—anti-inflammatory, antibacterial, antiseptic, anti-infectious, regenerative—healer for all types of skin, which can be used during pregnancy and on children. It is important, however, to check that the label clearly specifies "*angustifolia*," as this is the only type of lavender oil that is truly safe and effective for the skin.

In Chinese medicine, lavender is a slightly cooling oil with strong Qi-regulating properties. It promotes tissue repair, calms the mind, reduces fever and inflammation, and alleviates headaches, irritability, anxiety, and palpitations.

EMERGENCY ONLY: apply neat lavender oil on a burn, insect bite, or sting, but not on a large, open wound.

GOOD FOR: acne, dermatitis, dry and wet eczema, insect bites and stings, rashes, rosacea, sunburn, wounds, and burns (preventing scarring); regulating the fluid retention which causes puffy skin.

OTHER USES: calming and regulating the nervous system—headaches, migraine, and neuralgia; anti-spasmodic and sedative—relieves coughs and colds.

COMBINES WELL WITH: carrier oils—most, and particularly calendula, hazelnut, hypericum, macadamia nut, olive, sweet almond. For inflamed skin, combine with geranium, palmarosa, Roman chamomile, or rosewood essential oil.

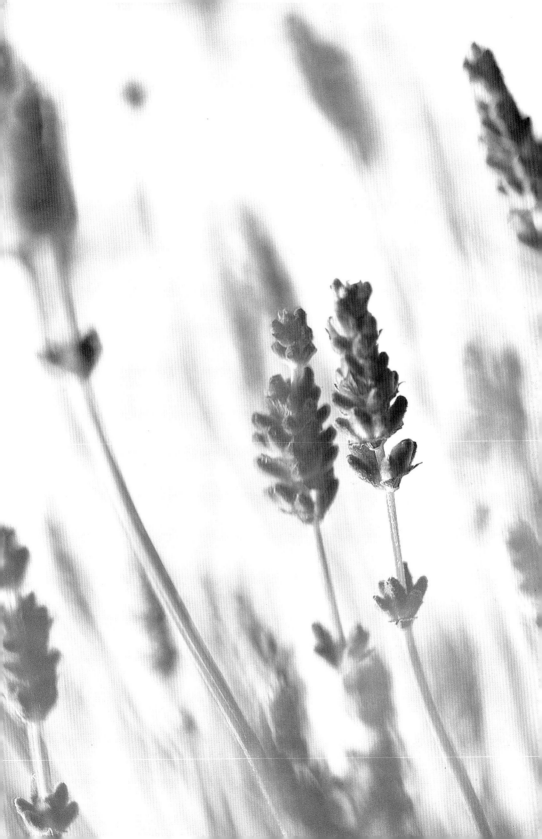

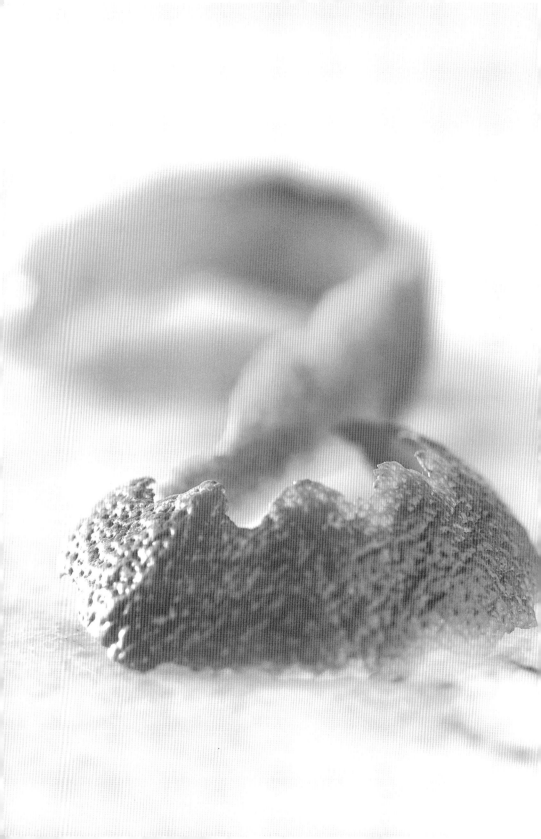

mandarin

A cold-pressed citrus oil obtained from the outer peel of the mandarin, this toning, antiseptic, fungicidal sweet oil is of great therapeutic value for the skin, particularly the oily type. It mixes well with other citrus oils, but it is slightly phototoxic, which means that if you use it and are then exposed to strong sunlight there can be some skin discoloration. So care should be taken with its use in summer.

In Chinese medicine, this oil is regarded as a slightly warm, yang oil, but with a sedating action. It is used extensively for digestive problems associated with irritability, for the insomnia caused by nervous tension, and for lifting the spirits, as well as for acne.

GOOD FOR: acne, oily skin, scars, pimples, stretch marks.

OTHER USES: anti-spasmodic—improves circulation of fluids; calming—good for stress; relieves digestive problems (including heartburn and colic; often recommended for children and pregnant women).

COMBINES WELL WITH: carrier oils—calendula, hazelnut, olive; essential oils—geranium, neroli.

myrrh

Obtained, like frankincense, by distillation from a resin, myrrh is derived from a species of commiphora tree native to the Red Sea region. It is a good antiseptic, fungicidal, anti-inflammatory, healing oil, with hormone-like properties, recommended for aging skin.

In Chinese medicine, myrrh is a warm, dry, yang oil. It is a stimulant and decongestant for the skin, can help to dispel colds and phlegm, and clear toxins. It is also used for reducing pain and swelling, and for ulcers.

GOOD FOR: chapped and cracked skin, cutaneous ulceration, mycosis (fungal infections), weeping eczema, wrinkles.

OTHER USES: amenorrhea (lack of periods), asthma, bronchitis, digestive problems, localized candidosis (thrush), sore throat.

COMBINES WELL WITH: carrier oils—apricot kernel, calendula, hypericum, jojoba, sweet almond; essential oils—cypress, frankincense, geranium, rosewood, tea tree.

neroli

This citrus oil, extracted by steam distillation from the flowers of the bitter orange (Citrus aurantium var. amara), was named after an Italian princess who used it daily as a perfume. Neroli, with its antibacterial, fungicidal, and healing properties, can be used for all types of skin. Although it is more costly than most of the oils listed, its therapeutic value on dry, aging skin and its beneficial action on spider and varicose veins or broken blood vessels in particular justify the expense.

In Chinese medicine, this oil has many similarities with mandarin. It is a slightly warm, yang oil with a strong calming action and is therefore used for stress, insomnia, anxiety, irritability, loss of appetite, and stomach pain. For the skin, neroli is useful for any condition that worsens with stress, and also where there is poor blood circulation.

GOOD FOR: dry, aging skin, problem skin (broken capillaries, seborrhea and pimples), scars, stretch marks, wrinkles.

OTHER USES: aids digestion; hypotensive (lowers blood pressure); remarkable dual effect on the central nervous system—antidepressant and calming, but also a gentle tonic to combat mental fatigue and poor concentration.

COMBINES WELL WITH: carrier oils—all those listed, especially apricot kernel, avocado, hazelnut; essential oils—all those listed, especially chamomile, geranium, lavender, rose otto. For dry, aging skin, choose a nourishing carrier such as apricot kernel, hazelnut, or sweet almond, add a small quantity of wheatgerm oil (and possibly borage oil), and combine a blend of chamomile, geranium, lavender, and neroli essential oils. For problem skin (see above), to a base of calendula and hazelnut with a little jojoba add a blend of neroli with cedarwood, clary sage, cypress, lavender, or rosewood.

niaouli

In the same family as the better-known tea tree (see page 65), niaouli is a very complex oil comprising over 100 constituent ingredients. As a strongly disinfectant, antiviral, antibacterial, and fungicidal oil, it is very useful for infected skin problems (especially if bacterial or fungal activity is evident or suspected), and as a powerful anti-inflammatory it also stops itching and allergic reactions. Niaouli scent is not to everybody's liking, so use only in small quantities, but as a good general oil suitable for all skin types and with no contra-indications it can even be applied neat to the skin for athlete's foot.

In Chinese medicine, niaouli is cooling, dry, and slightly yin. Its main actions are to clear toxins and reduce infection and inflammation. **GOOD FOR:** acne, dry and wet eczema, fungal infections (including athlete's foot), insect stings and bites, psoriasis, seborrheic dermatitis. **OTHER USES:** anti-inflammatory—rheumatism; helps to get rid of catarrh, colds, and flu; hormone-regulating—effective in men and women; improves poor blood circulation; relieves ear, nose, and throat infections and inflammation. **COMBINES WELL WITH:** carrier oils—all listed; essential oils—all listed.

palmarosa

From the same family as lemon grass and citronella and closely related to ginger grass, palmarosa is distilled from the leaves of a plant native to India and Pakistan. This is a must in skin care for all types of skin. A broad spectrum antimicrobial with a fungicidal action comparable to tea tree or niaouli, it is nonetheless very gentle to the skin, and its hydrating effect makes palmarosa valuable in any blend for ageing skin. Some aromatherapists recommend it in lip balms.

In Chinese medicine, this oil is cooling and more yin. It helps to regulate and balance Qi, reduces inflammation and fever, and promotes tissue repair. It is also said to calm the mind. **GOOD FOR:** acne, dermatitis, dry and wet eczema, dry skin, scars, wrinkles. **OTHER USES:** eases sinusitis and infections of the upper respiratory tract, ear, nose, and throat. **COMBINES WELL WITH:** carrier oils—apricot kernel, avocado, hazelnut, lime blossom, sweet almond; essential oils—cedarwood, cypress, geranium, rosewood, sandalwood.

patchouli

An extremely popular oil in India and tropical Asia, where it is often used to scent clothes to protect the wearer from insect bites and, even more importantly, to prevent the spread of disease, patchouli is distilled from the plant's fermented leaves. In addition to its insect repellent and antimicrobial qualities, it is a good anti-inflammatory and antiallergic oil with astringent properties, suitable for all types of skin.

In Chinese medicine, this oil is warm, drying, and yang. It is used to eliminate excess fluid and reduce inflammation.

GOOD FOR: acne, athlete's foot, dandruff, impetigo, inflammatory and allergic skin conditions, seborrheic dermatitis, spider, varicose, or broken veins, weeping eczema.

OTHER USES: aids digestion, antidepressant, effective insect repellent, prevents vomiting.

COMBINES WELL WITH: carrier oils—calendula, hazelnut, hypericum, jojoba, macadamia nut; essential oils—cedarwood, clary sage, cypress, geranium, lavender, neroli, palmarosa, rose otto, sandalwood. For an insect repellent, add sparingly to any blend.

rose otto

This is a very expensive oil, but it is money well spent. Available distilled from *Rosa damascena* (from Bulgaria) or *R. centifolia* (from Morocco or France), "otto" means obtained by steam distillation. Avoid the rose absolute (obtained by chemical extraction)—it is more likely to be of poor quality and may contain solvents that can cause allergic reactions. Used extensively for dry, aging skin, rose otto can help in many other dry skin conditions, and its astringent, antiseptic, anti-inflammatory properties are also recommended for sensitive skin. It can often help clear small, broken capillaries. A little goes a long way.

In Chinese medicine, rose otto is a slightly cool and yin oil. Astringent, stabilizing, and decongestant with moistening properties, this oil also benefits blood and regulates menstruation. It is also used to lift the spirits and relieve depression.

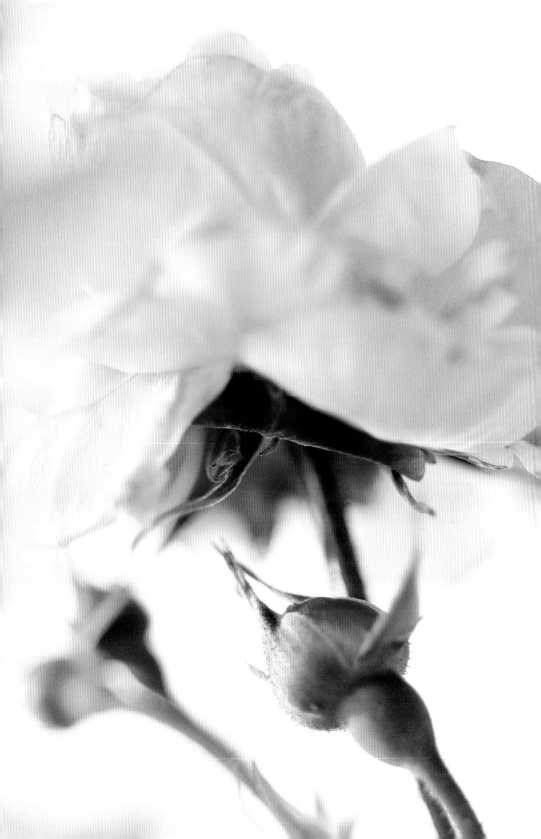

GOOD FOR: dryness, eczema, herpes, rashes, redness, rosacea, small broken capillaries, wrinkles.

OTHER USES: regulating hormones, stimulating the nervous system, and increasing sexual desires.

COMBINES WELL WITH: carrier oils—apricot kernel, avocado, borage, calendula, hazelnut, hypericum, lime blossom; essential oils—(for dry, aging skin) clary sage, geranium, lavender, palmarosa, and/or cypress, and (for sensitive skin) chamomile, lavender, patchouli, and sandalwood.

rosewood

Extracted by steam distillation from the wood chippings of Brazilian rosewood, this gentle, non-toxic, non-irritant oil is a good skin tonic, safe for any skin. Rosewood promotes skin regeneration and healing, being highly effective against a wide range of microorganisms, fungal infections, and viruses.

In Chinese medicine, this oil is gently cooling, slightly yin, and astringent. It aids the circulation of Qi and is calming.

GOOD FOR: acne, eczema, dermatitis, localized candidosis (thrush) in adults and babies, scars, wrinkles.

OTHER USES: headaches; baby rashes; nausea and stress-related conditions; upper respiratory tract infection in adults and babies.

COMBINES WELL WITH: carrier oils—all listed; essential oils—all listed.

sandalwood

One of the oldest perfumes in the world, the best sandalwood oil comes from India. Obtained by distillation from the wood of the tree, this is a very gentle oil, suitable for any type of skin. Its antiseptic, moisturizing properties are especially helpful for dry skin conditions.

In Chinese medicine, sandalwood is cool, yin, and astringent. It is a calming oil used for stress and depression; it aids circulation of Qi, vitalizes blood, moistens the skin, and alleviates night sweats, fever, and flushing.

GOOD FOR: acne, damaged skin, chapped or cracked skin, inflamed skin (including barber's rash, see below).

OTHER USES: antiemetic—nausea and mild diarrhea; calming and relaxing—

depression and insomnia; stimulating blood circulation—constricting small blood vessels; stimulating heart (mild).

COMBINES WELL WITH: carrier oils—apricot kernel, avocado, calendula, sweet almond; essential oils—geranium, jasmine, lavender, myrrh, niaouli, palmarosa, patchouli, rose otto, rosewood. Combine with lavender or rosewood for shaving rash (very effective).

tea tree

The leaves of the tea tree, native only to Australia, were already being eaten as a medicine by the Aboriginal people about 40,000 years ago. Distilled by steam extraction for a wide-spectrum antiseptic and anti-inflammatory oil, tea tree is exceptionally powerful in its bactericidal action and yet remarkably kind to all types of skin. A strongly scented oil, it is also an effective insect repellent.

In Chinese medicine, this is a cooling, slightly yin oil. It aids the circulation of Qi and blood, clears toxins, and reduces inflammation.

GOOD FOR: abscesses, boils, burns, cold sores, dandruff, fungal infections of feet and nails (most effective), herpes, infected acne and eczema, impetigo, insect bites, warts.

OTHER USES: stimulating the nervous system, heart, and immune system; fighting bronchitis, colds, ear, nose and throat infections, and flu.

COMBINES WELL WITH: carrier oils—calendula, hypericum, jojoba, macadamia nut; essential oils—chamomile, cypress, lavender, rosewood, sandalwood. To use as an insect repellent, simply add tea tree sparingly to any blend.

USING PRE-MIXED MASSAGE OILS

Many specialty aromatherapy companies are now offering high-quality massage oil blends of pure essential oils combined with one or several of the carrier oils mentioned in this book. While mixing your own oils is less expensive and quite easy, you may use one of these commercial blends if you are short on time or not inclined to mix your own. Just be sure to read the label carefully to find a blend that includes the carrier and essential oils best suited to your skin type. Also, perform a patch test first to avoid problems with potential allergic reactions.

carrier oils

	normal skin	dry skin	oily skin	combination skin	aging skin
apricot kernel	•••	•••••	•	••••	•••••
avocado	••	•••••	•	••	•••••
calendula	•••	•	•••••	•••	••
grapeseed	•••••	•••	••	••••	•
hazelnut	••••	••	••••	••••	•••
hypericum	•••	••	••••	•••	•••
jojoba	•	•••	••••	•••	•
lime blossom	••	•••	•	•••	•••••
macadamia nut	•	•••	••••	•••	•••
olive	•••••	•••••	•••••	•••••	•••••
sweet almond	•••••	••••	•••	•••••	••••
wheatgerm	••	•••••	•	•••	•••••
borage	••	•••	•	•	•••••
vitamin e	••	•••••	•	••	•••••

○ = no potency   • = low potency   ••••• = high potency

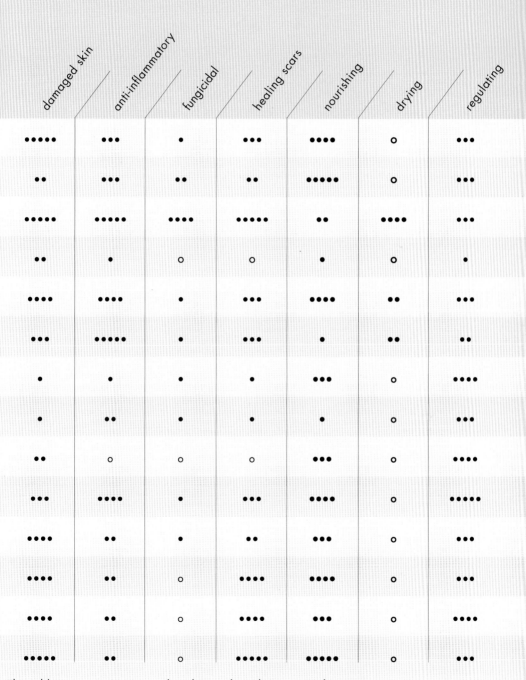

This table represents a personal evaluation based on practical experience.
Supplementary oils are listed in italic and can be added in small quantities to carrier oils (see page 47).

essential oils

	normal skin	dry skin	oily skin	combination skin	aging skin	damaged skin	toxicity in pregnancy	anti-inflammatory	antib...
cedarwood	••	•	••	••	••	•••••	•••	o	o
chamomile *german*	••	•	•••	•••	•••	•••	•	•••••	•••
chamomile *roman*	••	•	•••	•••	•••	•••	•	•••	•••
clary sage	••	•••	••	••	•••••	•	•••••	•	•
cypress	••	•	•••••	••	••••	•••••	o	o	•••
frankincense	••	••••	••	••	••••	•••••	o	•••	o
geranium	•••	•••••	•	•	••••	•••	o	•••	•••
jasmine	•••	•••	••	•••	••	•	o	o	•
juniper	•	•	•••	••	•	••	•••	•	••••
lavender	•••	••	•••••	••••	•••	•••••	o	•••	•••
mandarin	••	•	•••••	•••	•••	••	o	•	•
myrrh	••	•••	•••	•••	•••	••••	•	•••	•••
neroli	••	••••	•	••	••••	•••	o	••	•••
niaouli	•••	•••	•••	•••	•••	••	••	•••	••••
palmarosa	•••	•••	••	•••	•••	•••	o	••••	•••
patchouli	••	••	•••	•••	•••	•••	o	•••	•••
rose otto	••	•••	••	•••	•••••	•••	••	•••	••
rosewood	•••	•••	•••	•••	•••	•••	o	••	•••
sandalwood	•••	•••	••	•••	••	••	o	•	•
tea tree	••	••	•••	•••	••	•••	o	•••	•••••

o = no potency   • = low potency   ••••• = high potency

fungicidal	antiviral	hydrating	regulating/balancing	calming	stimulating	healing scars	astringent	photosensitivity	antiallergic
○	○	○	●●	●	●	●●●●	●●	○	○
●●	○	○	●	●●●●●	○	●	○	○	●●
●●	○	○	●	●●●●	○	○	○	○	●
○	○	●●	●●●●	●●●●	○	○	●	○	○
●●●	○	○	●●●●	●●●	●	●●●●	●●●●	○	○
○	○	○	●●●	●●●	●	●●●●	●●	○	○
●●●	●	●●●●	●●●●	●●●●	●	●	●●	○	●
○	○	●	●	●	●●●	○	●●	○	○
●	○	○	○	●	●●	●●●	●●●	○	○
●	●	○	●●●	●●●	○	●●●●	○	○	●●●
●	○	●	●●●	●●●●●	○	○	●●	●●●●	○
●●	●●	●	●●●	●●	●	●●●●	●	○	○
●●	●	●●	●●●	●●●	●	●●●	○	○	○
●●●	●●●●	●	●●	●	○	○	●	○	●
●●●	●●	●●	●●	●●	●	●●	●	○	●
●	○		●●	●	●●	●	●●	○	○
○	○	●●	●●●	●	●●●		●●	○	●
●●●	●●●	●	●●	●●●	●●	○	●●	○	●
○	○	●	●●●	●●	●●	○	●●	○	○
●●●●	●●●●	●	●	●	●●	○	○	○	○

This table represents a personal evaluation based on practical experience.

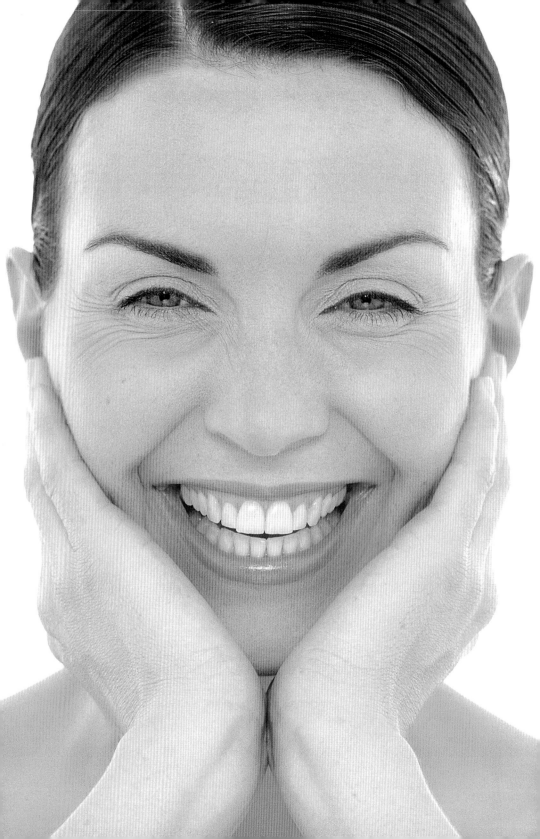

the
massage
program

You will be using fifteen different acupressure points in this program; most of them are paired, and all are on the face. The following section describes their positions and their specific effects, both on your face and, in some cases, on other parts of your body. Remember, as you consult the illustration, that unlike it, your face is three-dimensional. Learn to locate the points confidently before you begin to use the oils. You will know when you have found the right place because your skin will feel softer and a little sticky at each point. Press gently and you may feel a slight tingling sensation. (See page 125 for body pressure points that can be used to improve your general health and well-being.)

locating the acupressure points

TOP

T1: at top of nose, between eyebrows This point affects the vertical lines that appear between the eyebrows. It circulates Qi (see page 29) on the forehead, clears the eyes and nose, reduces any inflammation of the eyes, and is good also for relieving stress and depression.

T2: on forehead directly above T1 at hairline The forehead and scalp are affected by this point. In combination with T3 and T4, it can help fade the thin transverse lines that appear on the forehead. It is also good for relieving headaches.

T3: about ½–¾ in. (1cm.) each side of T2 These points work with T2 and T4 on transverse lines on the forehead. They also circulate Qi, regulate body fluids, and are effective for headache and sinus problems.

T4: on forehead, in hollow, about ½–¾ in. (1cm.) above middle of each eyebrow Along with T2 and T3, these help reduce frown lines and transverse lines on the forehead. They also relieve migraine and any redness, inflammation, or itching of the eyes.

SIDES

S1: on side of face, at end of each eyebrow Used in conjunction with S2, these act on the crow's feet that extend out toward the temples. They are also excellent points at which to alleviate tension headaches.

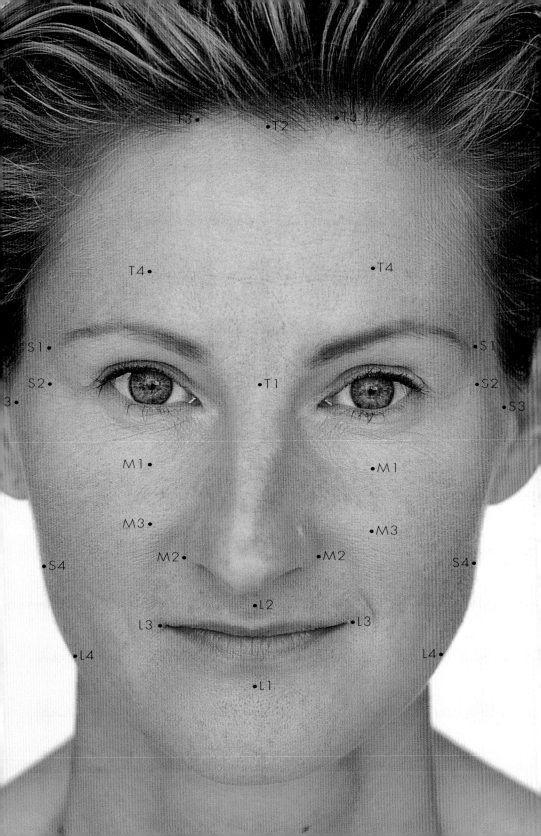

S2: on side of face, at corner of each eye The natural partners of S1; their effect is similar.

S3: approx. level with S2, but very close to each ear These points work upon the texture of the skin at the temples. They are also useful for earache and tinnitus (ringing in the ears), and release tension in the jaw.

S4: at each upper "angle" of jaw, in small hollow Important points, these affect the jawline and also tone the skin and muscles of the upper part of the neck.

MIDDLE
M1: on cheek ½–¾ in. (1cm.) below each eye in line with T4 Skin and muscle tone around the cheeks are affected by these points. They also act upon the sinuses and eliminate excess fluids or fatty deposits.

M2: at outer angle of each nostril These are important points for the deep wrinkles that appear between the nose and corners of the mouth. They can help to eliminate toxins, act on the sinuses or a blocked nose, and can also improve a poor sense of smell.

M3: ½–¾ in. (1cm.) directly below M1, at same level as M2 Found close to M1, these points are combined with M1, M2, and S3 to tone the skin and muscles of the cheeks.

LOWER
L1: between lower lip and chin, in line with tip of nose This important point for the whole face works specifically on the mouth and chin. It also stimulates the circulation of fluids around the mouth and cheeks as far as M1.

L2: between upper lip and base of nose The small wrinkles that appear around the mouth are reduced by this point. It can also clear the nose and eyes.

L3: at each end of mouth Used in conjunction with L1 and L2, these points firm the mouth. Combined with M1, M3, L4, and S4, they have a general toning effect on the entire face and the jawline. They can also eliminate small pimples or localized acne.

L4: at each lower "angle" of jaw These points should be used in conjunction with M3, L1, L3, and S4 to improve the shape of the jawline.

massage technique

Different parts of the sequence require different techniques. Sometimes you will use just the flat pad at the end of one finger (or thumb), sometimes the pads of your index, second, and third fingers placed together, side by side. Unless otherwise specified, the pressure is always firm.

There are two basic movements in the massage program. One is a rotating movement which travels slowly across the skin in a series of tiny spirals. The other is a simple, sliding movement, working upward, downward, or outward. On most occasions the remainder of your hand should rest very lightly on your face. In addition, you will be applying a pinching technique. Use the thumb and index finger lightly, but with enough strength to stimulate circulation. If your skin tone is pale, you should see a color change—to light pink—but take care not to bruise the skin. Pinching should be light when applied to the eyebrows and upper part of the face; much heavier when applied along the jawline.

USING YOUR BLENDED OIL

It is best to pour some of your blended oil (see pages 38–41) onto a small plate. You need so little on the pads of your fingers that this is a good way to avoid overload. It is easy enough to add a little more if you find that your fingers are sticking to your skin. Take care not to get oil in your eyes. (See pages 40–41 for more on safety precautions.)

PREPARING FOR MASSAGE

A peaceful atmosphere is vital to the success of this program, so do your best to approach it in a relaxed way. Before you start, make sure that you have everything you need in front of or beside you as you stand or sit comfortably in front of a mirror—a little of your blended oil poured onto a plate, a wet cloth to dampen your skin (it helps the mixture to emulsify and penetrate more easily), and a terrycloth and/or elastic band to make sure that all your hair is away from your face. Do the massage on clean skin once or twice a day as indicated in the six-week plan for your skin type (see pages 98–103). It takes approx. 14 minutes. Apart from stimulating blood circulation and Qi, it is very effective in relieving the tensions of a demanding day.

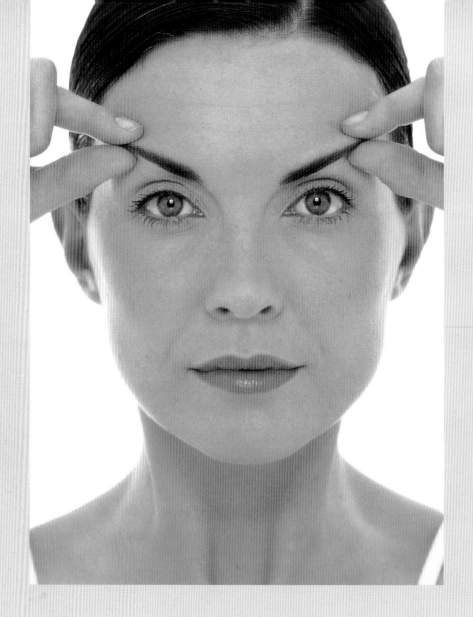

Warm-up sequence

1 Using your thumbs and index fingers and starting at the top of the nose between the eyes, pinch gently but firmly all along each eyebrow. Continue the action as far as possible along the temples, toward the tip of each ear.
2 Do the same pinching movement, starting from the center of the chin and this time working slowly along the jawline and up to the base of the ear. Do steps 1 and 2 three times.
3 Dampen your skin with the wet cloth. Then dip the pads of your fingers lightly into your oil and gently rub your palms together to spread it.

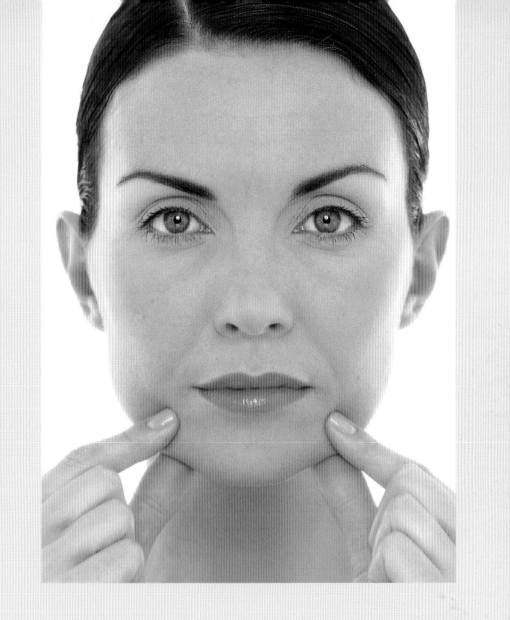

All the steps that follow should be carried out on both sides of the face simultaneously. Step 1 is an important sequence, used to begin and end your 20-step massage. Purely practically, it spreads the oil over your face. But it also centers and stills you before and after the massage, and helps the energy to flow.

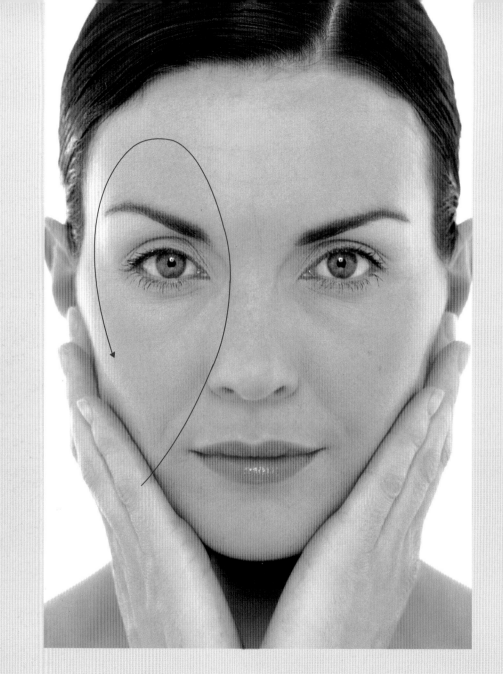

Position your palms on your jawline so that your fingertips rest lightly on your cheekbones and pause for a beat or two. With light pressure, slide the pads of your first three fingers in a sweeping movement up along your nose, through the middle of your forehead, and down along your hairline. Continue on down your temples to meet at the middle of your jawbone.

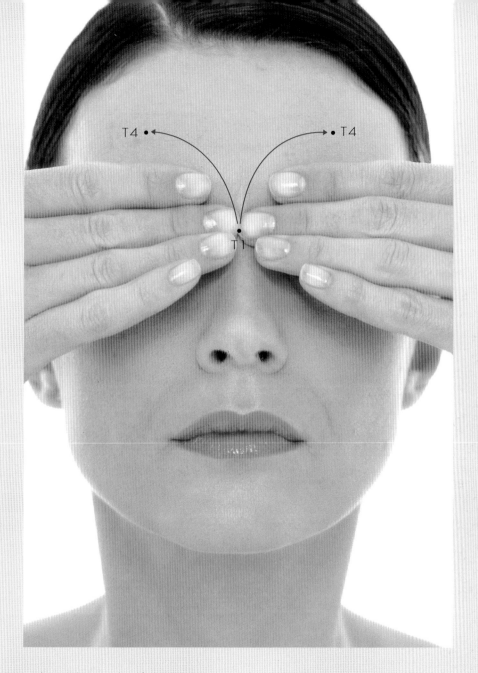

T4 •←   →• T4

T1

Place the pads of the same three fingers at the T1 pressure point
and slide them upward to T4. Do this three times.
(This step can help relieve the tension that causes us to frown.)

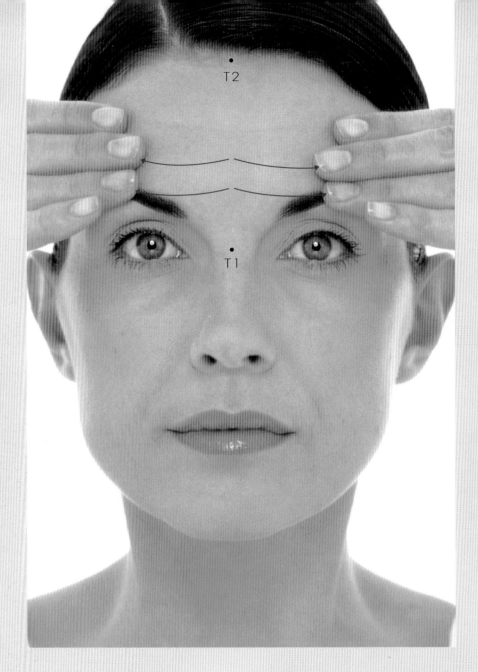

Positioning the pads of the same three fingers at the base of your central frown line, between T1 and T2, slide your fingers out toward your temples, smoothing the skin as you go. Do this three times.

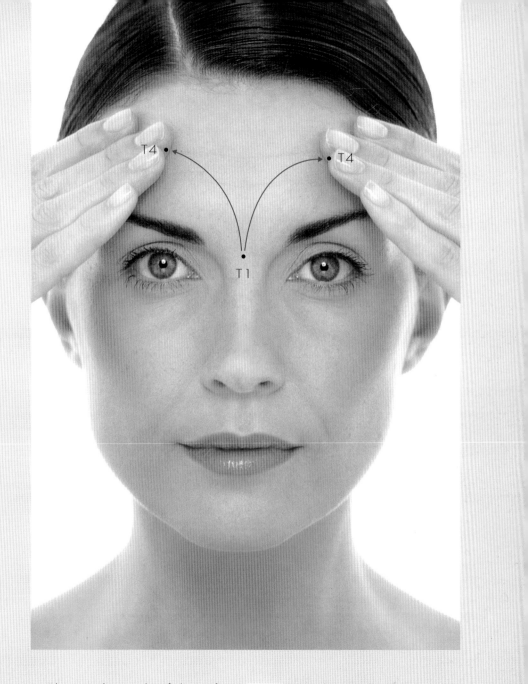

Placing the pads of these fingers at T1, make small, spiraling
movements outward to T4. Do this three times.

4

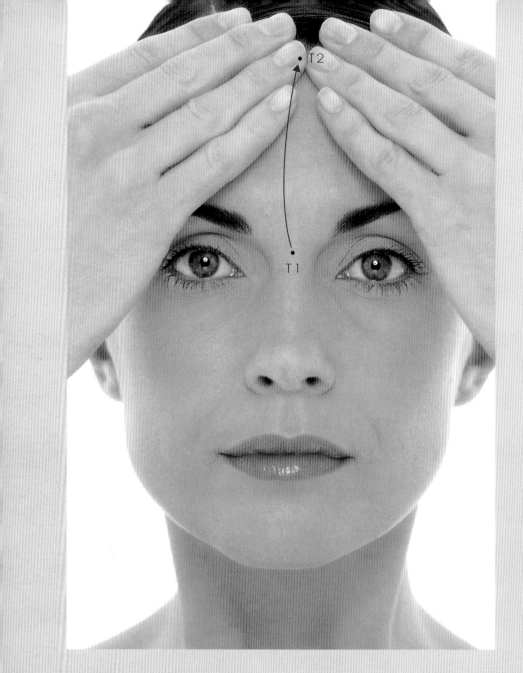

Slide the same three fingers up the central frown line from T1 to T2.
Do this three times.

5

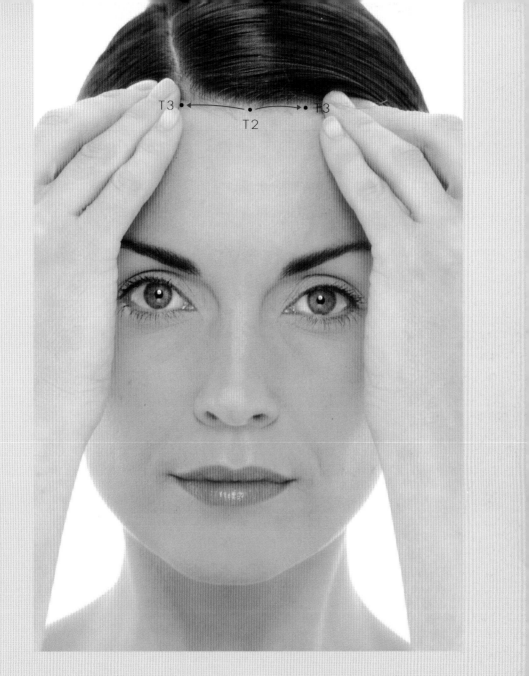

T3 •←——— • ——→• T3
T2

Place the pads of the same three fingers at T2 and make little spiraling movements along the hairline to T3 and then all the way down to the temples. Do this three times, and then continue the same movement to S1, to S2, and finally to S3. (This step is a useful way to prevent headaches.)

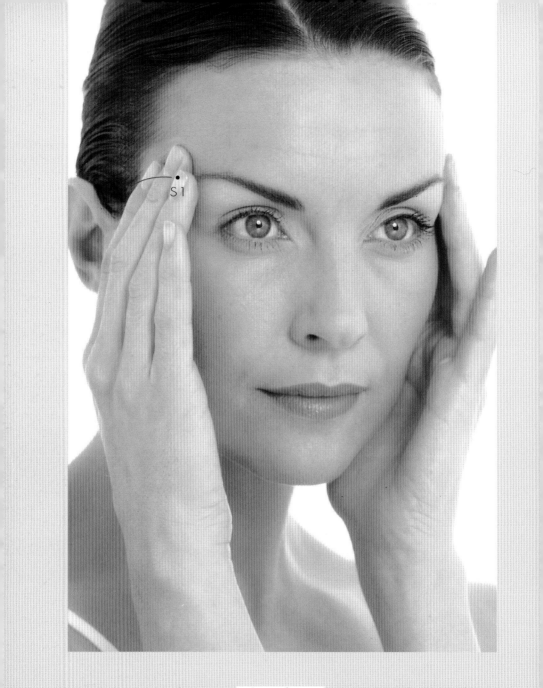

With the pads of the same three fingers at S1, spiral outward to
the hairline, level with the top of each ear. Do this three times.
Now slide your fingers over the same area instead of making
spirals. Do this three times.

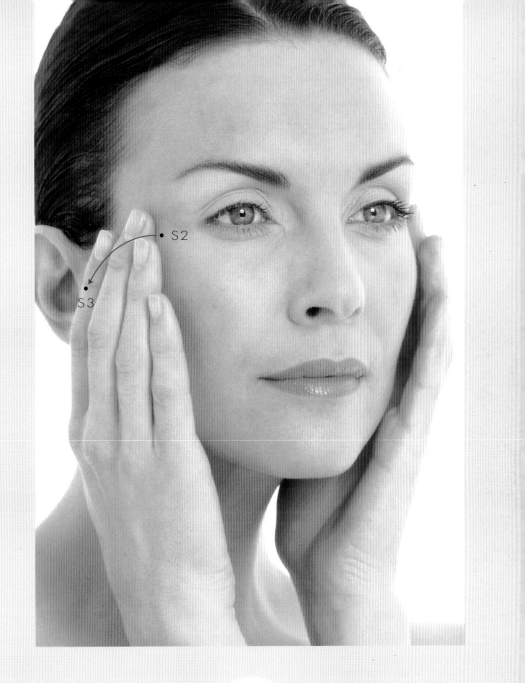

Using the same movements (first spiraling, then sliding), massage from S2 to S3, taking care to apply less pressure, so that you do not stretch the skin. Do each movement three times.

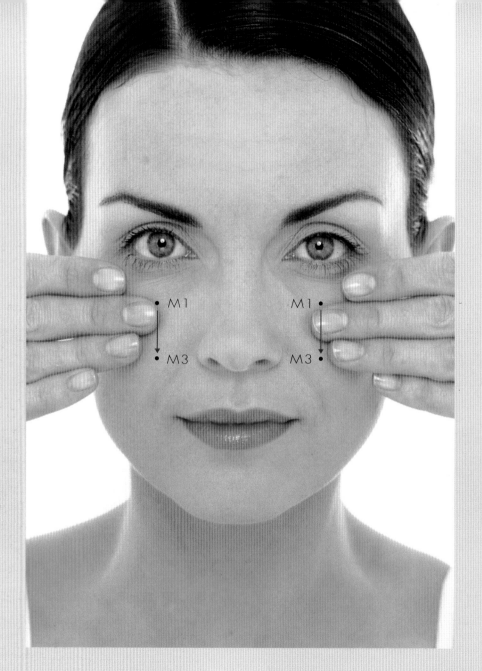

M1 • M1 •

• M3 • M3

Place the pads of these three fingers at M1 and spiral gently down to M3, using the tips of your middle fingers only. Do this three times. Then repeat another three times, now sliding all three fingers down to M3.

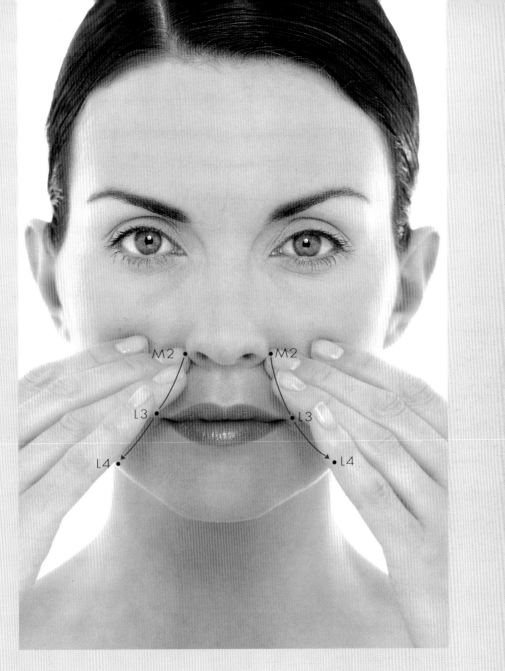

Positioning the pads of these three fingers at M2, spiral downward
and outward to L3 and then to L4, again using just the tips of
your middle fingers. Do this three times. Then repeat three times,
now sliding all three fingers. (Steps 9 and 10 will help to tone
the muscles around the cheekbones, as well as relieving
congested sinuses.)

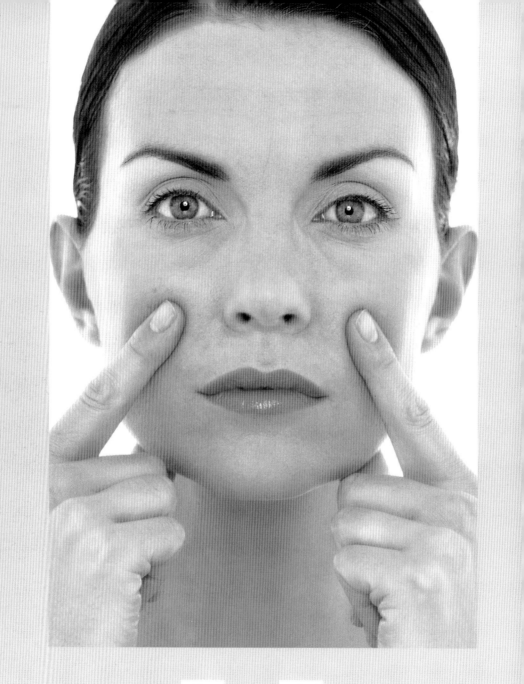

Just under your cheekbones, level with the middle of your eyes, there are two small indentations. Place the pads of your index fingers here and press gently upward onto the bone, hold for a few seconds, and then release. Do this three times.

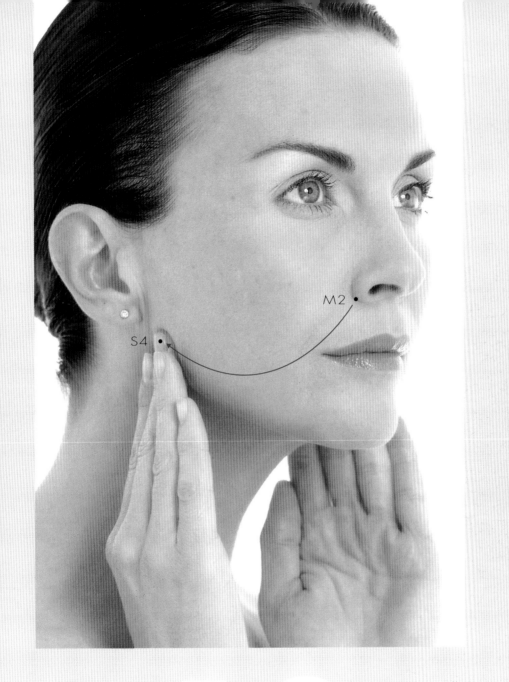

With the pads of your first three fingers again at M2, use small, deep spiraling movements to massage under the cheekbones and toward S4. Do this three times.

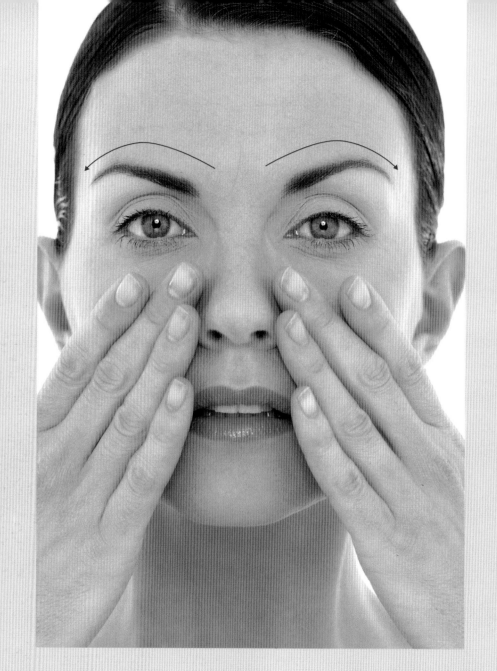

Place one hand on each side of your nose, palms together. [In this photograph the palms have not yet joined] With firm, even pressure, move each hand outward toward the temples and the ears—during this movement the palms of your hands should be pressing against the lower part of your face. Do this three times.

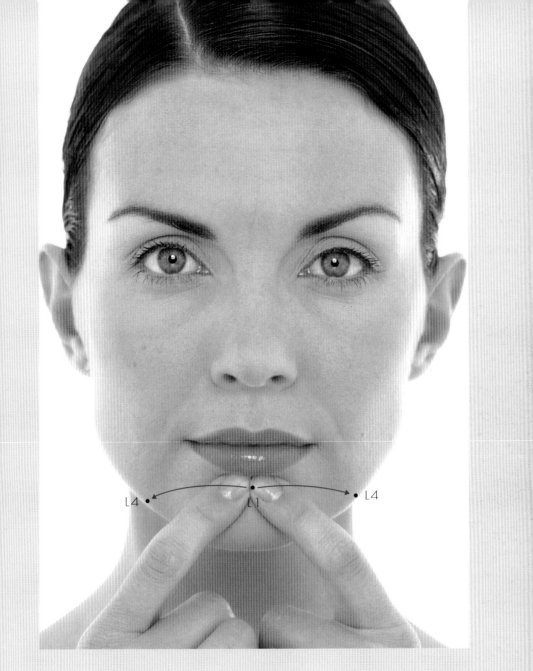

L4 •   • L1   • L4

Using the pads of either your index or second fingers, massage from L1 to L4, using small, deep rotating movements. Do this three times. (This sequence will release toxins and ease tension around the mouth and jaw.)

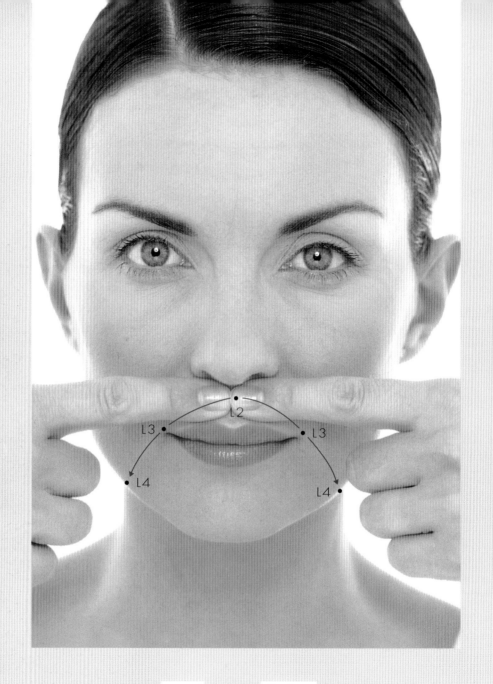

Slide the pads of your index or middle fingers from L2 down to L3 and out to L4. Do this three times. Repeat another three times, now using small, deep rotating movements.

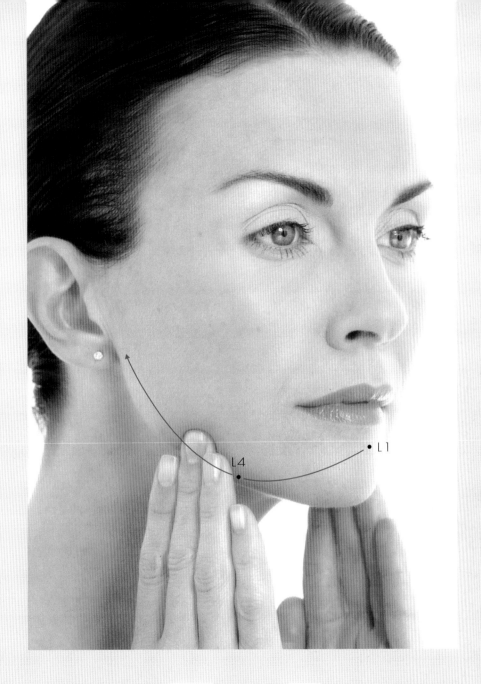

Place the pads of your index or middle fingers on L1 and slide them out to L4. Do this three times. Then rest the pads of all three fingers on the jawline, beneath the mouth, and make slow, spiraling movements outward along the jaw to the lobes of your ears. Do this three times.

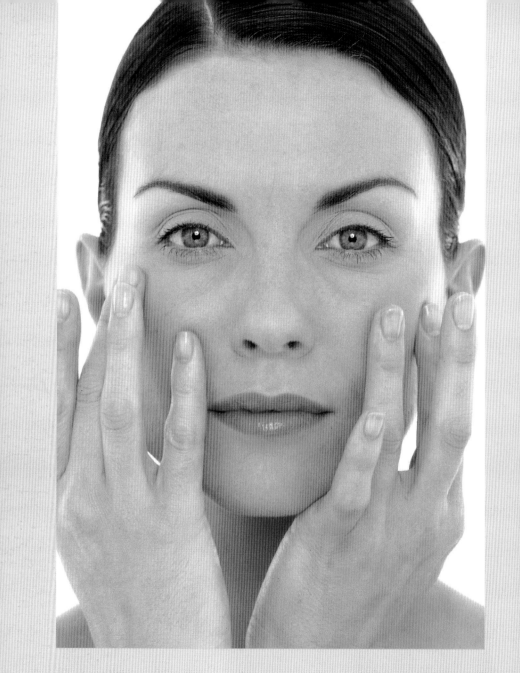

Using just the very tips of your fingers, tap featherlightly all over your forehead and cheeks. (This action tones the tissues and gently stimulates the flow of blood to these areas.)

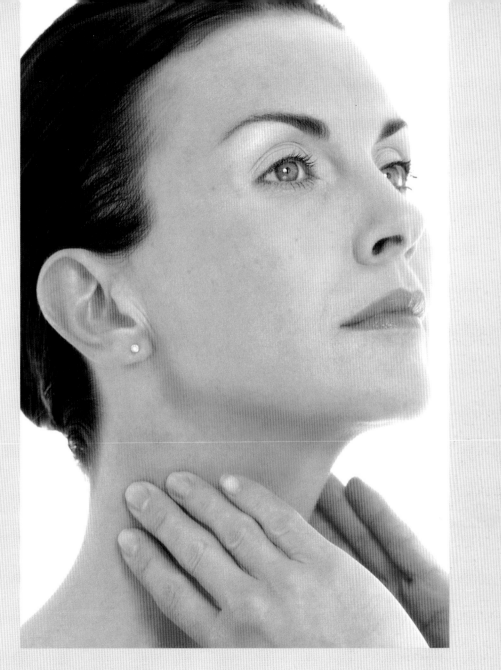

Place your hands on each side of the base of your neck, with your fingertips pointing away from your chin. Using the flat part of your fingers, make larger spiraling movements over the big muscle at each side, traveling up as far as your hairline. Do this three times. (This step can reduce the tension that builds up from sitting, driving, or talking for a long time.)

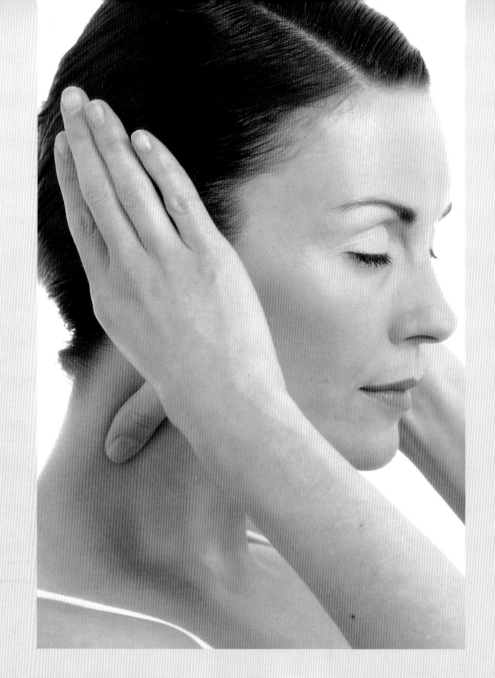

Rest the palms of your hands on your ears with your thumbs
pointing downward. Use both thumbs to massage with broad,
spiraling movements from your throat to the back of your neck.
Do this three times.

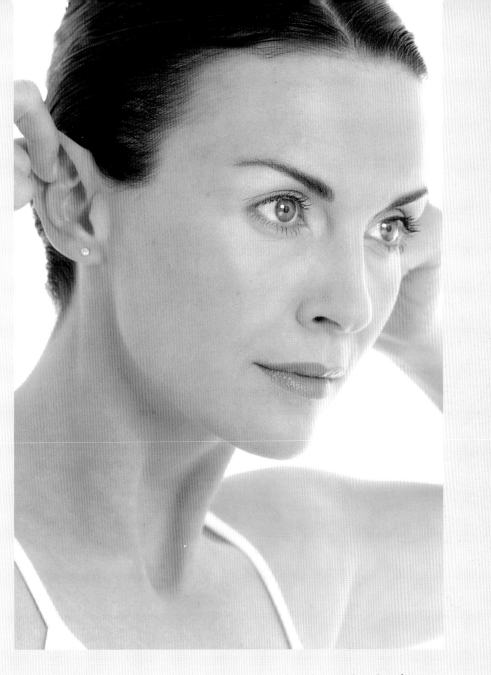

Hold the tops of your ears between your thumbs and index fingers and make little pinching movements all around the edge until you reach the point where the lobes meet the face. (There are many pressure points on and in the ear that connect to the whole body, so working the ear is important.) Repeat steps 1–20 and then complete the massage with step 1.

six-week plans for a younger face

These six-week plans have been developed to suit the five basic skin types and can be adapted for any existing skin condition. Each one sets out a daily schedule for the massage program (see pages 70–97) and proposes a detailed sequence of skin-care suggestions, such as steaming the skin or specialized face masks and lotions, designed to support and enhance the main objectives of each plan.

It is important to be consistent and patient, as six weeks is a relatively short time to get good results for your skin. You will probably need longer than this to notice a major difference, and ideally you should carry on doing the massage technique at least once a day all year long as a general maintenance program.

normal skin

If you are lucky enough to have good skin, all you need to do as well as your daily massage program is a regular, gentle routine to remove dead cells and impurities and nourish your skin to keep it healthy.

To enhance this six-week plan it would be helpful to reduce your alcohol consumption, stop smoking, increase exercise in the open air, and, if needed, go on a gentle weight-reduction diet.

1 Massage morning and evening, using a normal-skin oil recipe (see page 36).
To cleanse Gently steam your face once this week, using a chamomile and rosemary herb mix (see page 121).
To tone Not necessary daily, but use rosewater (see page 126) after steaming.

2 Massage morning and evening, using an appropriate oil recipe (see page 36).
To nourish Apply a fruit mask (see pages 112–16) once this week, choosing fresh apricots, blackcurrants, or strawberries.
To tone Apply almond lotion (see page 112) every day after massage. Alternatively, apply a little rosewater.

3 Massage morning and evening, using an appropriate oil recipe (see page 36).
To nourish Apply a fruit mask once this week as in week 2.
To tone Apply either almond lotion or rosewater as in week 2.

4 Massage once a day, using an appropriate oil recipe (see page 36).
To cleanse Apply a clay and spirulina mask (see page 110, To nourish normal skin) once this week.
To tone Apply almond lotion once a day after massage.

5 Massage once a day, using an appropriate oil recipe (see page 36).
To cleanse Give your skin a rest from deep cleansing for a week.
To tone Apply either almond lotion or rosewater once a day after massage.

6 Massage morning and evening, using an appropriate oil recipe (see page 36).
To nourish Apply a honey mask (see page 119, For normal skin) once this week.
To tone Apply almond lotion after the mask and every day after massage.

dry skin

To support this six-week plan you need to cool and hydrate your skin. It is advisable to reduce your alcohol consumption as much as possible, and, if you smoke, to try to stop. Changes in diet can help too—include more carrots, spinach, dried apricots, brazil nuts, fresh fruit, wheatgerm, fortified breakfast cereals, olive oil, and fish.

After week 6, continue to do the massage program once a day at least. Apply a nourishing fruit mask (see pages 112–16) once a week, and occasionally make a clay and spirulina mask (see page 110, To revitalize dry skin).

1 Massage morning and evening, using a dry-skin oil recipe (see page 36).
To nourish Apply an avocado mask (see page 115, For dry skin) twice this week.
To tone Apply rosewater (see page 126) after the mask and every day after massage.

2 Massage morning and evening, using an appropriate oil recipe (see page 36).
To nourish Apply a honey and yogurt mask (see page 119, For dry skin 1) to your face once this week.
To tone Apply rosewater as in week 1.

3 Massage morning and evening, using an appropriate oil recipe (see page 36).
To nourish Apply a honey and egg white mask (see page 119, For dry skin 2) to your face once this week.
To tone Apply rosewater as in week 1.

4 Massage morning and evening, using an appropriate oil recipe (see page 36).
To nourish Apply an avocado mask twice this week as in week 1.
To tone Apply rosewater as in week 1.

5 Massage morning and evening, using an appropriate oil recipe (see page 36).
To nourish Apply an almond mask (see page 112) once this week.
To tone Apply rosewater as in week 1.

6 Massage morning and evening, using an appropriate oil recipe (see page 36).
To nourish Apply a honey and egg white mask once this week as in week 3.
To tone Apply rosewater as in week 1.

oily skin

To support this six-week plan you need to cleanse your skin regularly and close the pores. Cut down on alcohol, stop smoking, and avoid pork and dairy products as much as possible. Increase your intake of fresh vegetables, fortified breakfast cereals, wheatgerm, brown rice, and olive oil, and take a daily multivitamin supplement including vitamin B complex, selenium, and zinc. If dieting, opt for a low-fat, low-calorie approach.

After week 6, repeat the six-week plan. Then continue the massage once a day. During winter and spring, alternate steaming and a clay mask (as for week 1) once every two weeks.

1 Massage morning and evening, using an oily-skin oil recipe (see page 37).
To cleanse Steam your face with lavender and chamomile herbs (see page 121) and (three days later) use a clay and witchhazel mask (see page 108, To clean oily skin).
To tone Apply rosewater (see page 126) after steaming, the mask, and every day after massage.

2 Massage morning and evening, using an appropriate oil recipe (see page 37).
To cleanse Gently steam your face once this week as in week 1.
To tone Apply rosewater after steaming and every day after massage.

3 Massage morning and evening, using an appropriate oil recipe (see page 37).
To cleanse Apply a clay and witch hazel mask as in week 1 twice this week at three-day intervals.
To tone Apply rosewater after the mask and every day after massage.

4 Massage morning and evening, using an appropriate oil recipe (see page 37).
To cleanse Gently steam your face once this week as in week 1.
To tone Apply rosewater as in week 2.

5 Massage morning and evening, using an appropriate oil recipe (see page 37).
To nourish Apply a honey and cucumber mask (see page 120, For oily skin) to your face once this week.
To tone Apply rosewater as in week 3.

6 Massage morning and evening, using an appropriate oil recipe (see page 37).
To cleanse Steam your face once this week as in week 1 and (three days later) gently clean once using a honey and cucumber mask as in week 5.
To tone Apply rosewater as in week 1.

combination skin

To enhance this six-week plan, it is important to clean and hydrate the skin well. Stop smoking and cut down on alcohol. Reduce your consumption of dairy products, pork, and anything spicy, eat more foods rich in vitamins A and B (spinach, watercress, carrots, leafy green vegetables, brown rice, liver, and fish, for example) and use olive oil for cooking and salad dressings. Take a multivitamin supplement that includes vitamin B complex and zinc daily.

After week 6, continue the massage once a day, and use a mixture of equal quantities of almond lotion (see page 112) and rosewater (see page 126) to tone your skin every day after massage.

Massage morning and evening, using a combination-skin oil recipe (see page 37).
To cleanse Gently steam your face once this week by using the chamomile and rosemary herb mix (see page 121).
To tone Apply rosewater (see page 126) after steaming and every day after massage.

Massage morning and evening, using an appropriate oil recipe (see page 37).
To cleanse Gently steam your face once this week as in week 1.
To tone Apply rosewater after steaming and a lemon, rosewater, and witch hazel lotion (see page 116) every day after massage.

Massage morning and evening, using an appropriate oil recipe (see page 37).
To nourish Apply an avocado and egg mask (see page 115, For combination skin) once.
To tone Apply rosewater after the mask and the toning lotion as in week 2.

Massage morning and evening, using an appropriate oil recipe (see page 37).
To cleanse Apply a clay and spirulina mask (see page 110, To revitalize combination skin) twice this week, the second two days after the first.
To tone Apply rosewater after the mask and the toning lotion as in week 2.

Massage morning and evening, using an appropriate oil recipe (see page 37).
To nourish Apply an almond mask (see page 112) once this week.
To tone Apply rosewater after the mask, and a freshly pressed grape lotion (see page 116) every day after massage.

Massage morning and evening, using an appropriate oil recipe (see page 37).
To nourish Apply an avocado and egg mask once this week as in week 3.
To tone Apply rosewater after the mask and

aging skin

If your skin shows signs of aging and is often dry, you need to hydrate, nourish, and tone it well. To enhance this six-week plan, cut down on alcohol as much as possible and stop smoking. Eat more carrots, spinach, dried apricots, brazil nuts, fresh fruit, wheatgerm, fortified breakfast cereals, olive oil, and fish.

After week 6 continue the massage once a day. Make a nourishing fruit mask twice a week (see pages 112–16), and use almond lotion (see page 112), clary sage hydrosol or rosewater (see page 126) every day after massage to tone. Use cotton ball and cornflower hydrosol compresses for the area around the eyes.

1 Massage once a day, using a mature-skin oil recipe (see page 37).

To nourish Apply an avocado, honey, and egg mask (see page 115, For aging skin) to your face twice this week.

To tone Apply rosewater (see page 126) after the mask and every day after massage.

2 Massage once a day, using an appropriate oil recipe (see page 37).

To nourish Apply a honey and yogurt mask (see page 119, For dry skin 1) to your face twice during this week.

To tone Apply rosewater as in week 1.

3 Massage morning and evening, using an appropriate oil recipe (see page 37).

To nourish Apply a pollen mask (see page 120) once this week.

To tone Apply a freshly pressed grape lotion (see page 116) to your face every evening after massage.

4 Massage morning and evening, using an appropriate oil recipe (see page 37).

To nourish Apply a honey and yogurt mask as in week 2.

To tone Apply rosewater after the mask and every day after massage.

5 Massage morning and evening, using an appropriate oil recipe (see page 37).

To nourish Apply an almond mask (see page 112) once this week.

To tone Apply rosewater after the mask and every day after massage.

6 Massage morning and evening, using an appropriate oil recipe (see page 37).

To nourish Apply a pollen mask as in week 3 and three days later a clay and parsley mask (see page 110, For mature neck).

To tone Apply rosewater after clay mask, two parts witch hazel to one part rosewater around eyes daily, and grape lotion as in week 3.

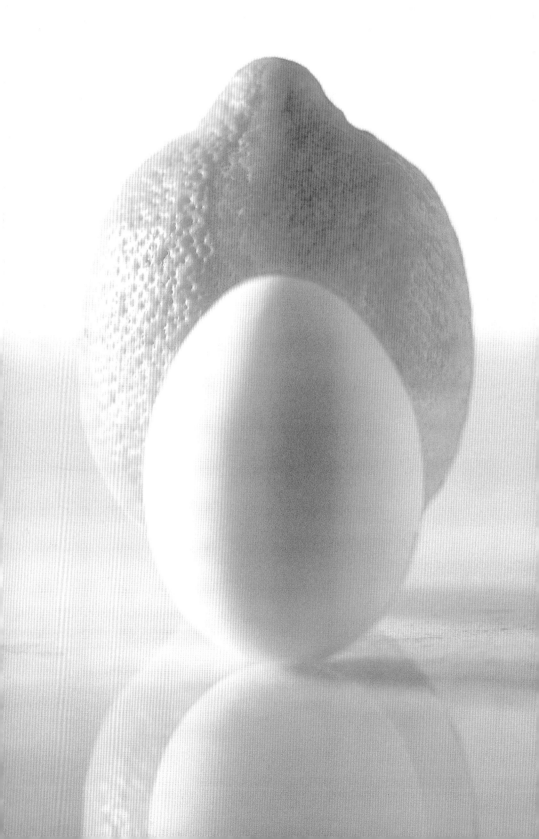

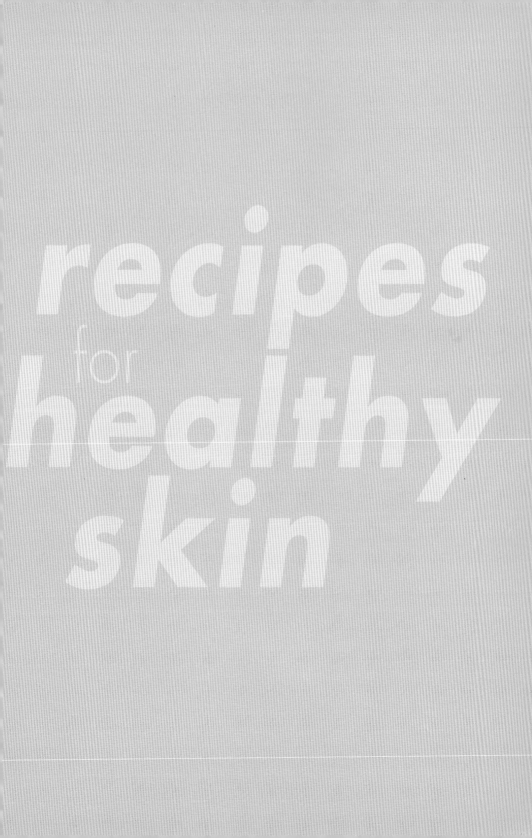

recipes for healthy skin

This resource section provides you with a whole range of optional treatments you can draw upon to use with the massage program (see pages 70–97) and the oils that suit your skin type.

The major part contains recipes designed to cleanse, tone, or nourish the skin. The six-week plans on pages 98–103 will give you some guidance on how to make the most of them. Always use the recommendations in your plan as a starting point.

Almost all the ingredients included can be listed in five very simple categories—clay, nuts and fruit, herbs, bee products, and eggs and dairy products. All of them and the techniques described can be tried safely, provided you follow the recommendations given. Some have been used for over a thousand years; many are employed in commercial products today, disguised by modern technology. It is easy to spend a small fortune on expensive cosmetics, not realizing that many of the natural agents included are available at a fraction of the cost in supermarkets or health-food stores and can be used to make healthful, simple alternative treatments.

On pages 122–24 you will find helpful advice on eating for healthy skin. Poor diet certainly contributes to, and may even accelerate, the process of aging. Even relatively minor deficiencies have long-term consequences, so it makes sense to remember the indispensable part that vitamins play in maintaining healthy skin.

The short list of additional acupressure points given on page 125 are all on the body. Used regularly, they can have a remarkable effect on your general sense of well-being, as well as (in some cases) contributing extra benefits to the look of your skin.

clay

Among the variety of natural ingredients that can be used to improve the skin, clay is probably the most effective. Used alone or mixed with other substances, clay can clean, detoxify, tone, and nourish any type of skin. It is cheap, versatile, and extremely simple to use—all facts that have not escaped the manufacturers of cosmetics, who offer at greatly inflated prices a variety of clay-based masks for rejuvenation.

Clay is a sediment composed of hydrated aluminum silicate and created by the slow erosion of granite. Various minerals, such as oxide of iron, salts, calcium, and trace elements, in varying proportion alter its therapeutic qualities and color.

The healing properties of clay are well established. Thousands of years ago, the ancient Egyptians were singing the praises of clay as a medicine and for the skin. The Chinese, Greeks, Romans, and early peoples of the Indian subcontinent all knew its excellent properties and used it both internally and externally.

It is an antiseptic, scientifically proven to be active against a wide range of microorganisms. It can draw out impurities from the deeper layers of the skin. It promotes healing and regeneration by helping to regulate fluid metabolism within the skin. As well as being anti-inflammatory, analgesic, and astringent, it also does not cause allergic reactions.

CHOOSING THE CLAY

Many clay (or kaolin) products are now available in health stores and pharmacies. To make good masks you need very fine white or green clay. If you buy one of the cheaper, coarser products, break it down in a blender. The best way to test the texture is to try a little on your tongue: it should not feel gritty. White clay is the more neutral and preferable for normal or combination skin. Green clay has a stronger therapeutic action and is more drying, so use it for oily skin.

USING CLAY MASKS

To be effective, a clay mask must be applied at least once a week. However, care must be taken when using clay masks on a dry skin. It can still be useful to remove toxins and dead cells regularly, but it is important to add a hydrating substance to the mix (essential oil, herbs, or olive oil, for example), and the mask should be removed as soon as you feel the skin begin to "pull." The basic recipe on the following page explains the principles of making and using a clay mask. In practice— using the recipes recommended in the six-week plans (see pages 98–103) and experimenting for yourself—you will be adding or substituting various ingredients for their extra nourishing or toning effects.

basic clay mask

Measure 2 to 3 tablespoons of your chosen clay into a glass or ceramic bowl and add about 3 tablespoons of bottled or spring water—enough to cover the clay by about ¼ in. (5mm.). It is important to use a water low in minerals. Do not use tap water.

Leave without stirring for 1 hour if possible (30 minutes at least). Stirring too soon affects the consistency of the mask, making it sticky and more difficult to apply. It is always easier to add a small amount of clay to a mix that is too thin than more water to a paste that is too thick.

Once you begin to stir, you are aiming for the consistency of yogurt, a smooth paste that can be applied without problems. If too liquid, it will not stick to the skin; if too thick, it will not be supple enough to penetrate deep into the skin. Adjust by adding a little more clay if necessary.

Use the tips of your fingers to apply the mask gently in thin layers to your face and/or neck, starting from the center of the forehead and working outward. Avoid the area around the eyes (see page 110).

Allow to dry naturally. At this stage avoid talking, smiling, or any other movement that will cause cracks to appear. When the mask is almost completely dry, rinse off with bottled or spring water, or rosewater (see Hydrosols, page 126) and pat the skin dry with cotton balls.

BOOSTING THE BASIC MIX

The following recipes are based upon the basic clay mask recipe above. Ingredients are added or substituted in the basic mix to enhance specific effects, so follow the indications and instructions carefully, referring to the basic method above.

To clean oily skin

Use green clay and substitute 2 to 3 tablespoons witch hazel (see Hydrosols, page 126) for the bottled water. Rinse and apply a little rosewater (also see Hydrosols).

To revitalize

Mix 1 tablespoon spirulina very thoroughly into your chosen clay before adding the bottled or spring water. For a perfectly smooth paste, use a blender. Spirulina (otherwise known as blue-green algae) is available in powder form from most health-food stores.

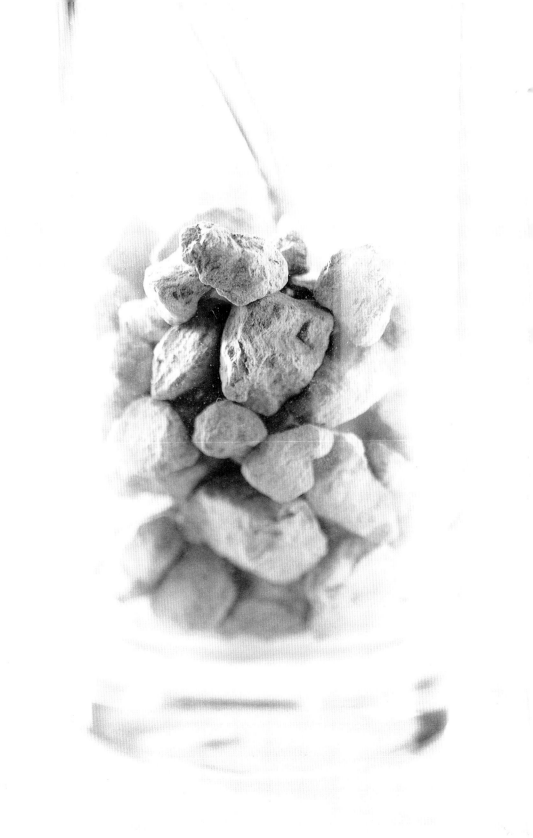

TO NOURISH NORMAL SKIN

Adding 1 tablespoon spirulina (see recipe above) to 2 tablespoons white clay, use almond lotion (see page 112) instead of bottled or spring water. You can also add 1 to 2 drops of one essential oil chosen from the supplementary list on page 47, if you wish—stir in before the lotion.

TO REVITALIZE DRY SKIN

Mix 1 tablespoon spirulina (see above) and 2 to 3 tablespoons white clay. Using a blender, process 1 to 2 carrots—enough to produce 2 tablespoons fresh carrot juice—and substitute for bottled or spring water.

TO REVITALIZE COMBINATION SKIN

Add 1 tablespoon spirulina (see above) to 2 tablespoons green clay and stir in 1 tablespoon olive oil, mixing well. Substitute rosewater (see Hydrosols, page 126) for bottled or spring water.

MASK FOR AREA AROUND EYES (ALL SKIN TYPES)

Mix 2 teaspoons of your chosen clay with 3 teaspoons witch hazel or cornflower water (see Hydrosols, page 126). Leave on for 10 minutes. Rinse off carefully with bottled or spring water, using cotton balls, and tone with a mixture of two parts rosewater (see Hydrosols) and one part witch hazel.

MASK FOR MATURE NECK

Add 2 tablespoons chopped fresh parsley to 2 tablespoons of your chosen clay, and stir in 1 tablespoon olive oil and 1 tablespoon wheatgerm oil. Then add 2 tablespoons witch hazel (see Hydrosols, page 126) instead of bottled or spring water, and mix immediately. Leave on for 35 minutes.

adding juices and purées

You can add fresh fruit or vegetable purées or juices to clay for a mask with even more specific therapeutic action. To nourish and tone tired, damaged skin of any type, use apricot, avocado, banana, carrot, cherry, cucumber, potato, or tomato. Use dandelion to detoxify and reduce inflammation on damaged skin, and to lighten freckles; grape to tone all types of skin (mixing 1 tablespoon wheatgerm carrier oil into your chosen clay before the juice); lemon to tone, disinfect, close pores, and eliminate pimples and blackheads on oily skin; parsley to tone and revitalize aging or damaged skin, and to lighten freckles; and watercress to reduce inflammation and revitalize damaged skin.

TO JUICE

Using a juicer or blender, extract about 3 tablespoons of juice from your chosen fruit, and add to 2 tablespoons of the appropriate clay, substituting for bottled or spring water in the basic recipe (see page 108). There is no need to leave it to "sit" before stirring.

TO PURÉE

Using a blender, process enough of your chosen fruit or vegetable to obtain 3 tablespoons of purée, and mix with just 1 tablespoon of the appropriate clay to make a smooth paste; add a little more clay if the mixture is too runny.

adding dried herbs

You can also add powdered medicinal herbs to your clay mix. One teaspoon of the dried plant is usually enough—dried herbs are very concentrated. Among the dried herbs easily available are several worth trying: birch, coltsfoot, or yarrow for chronic inflammation; burdock or plantain for eczema or acne; marshmallow just for eczema; horsetail or nettle for dermatitis; and comfrey for regeneration. You can use any of them fresh if you are lucky enough to find them: 1 to 2 tablespoons, well chopped, should be enough.

TO MAKE A MASK

Add 1 teaspoon dried herbs to 2 tablespoons clay and then follow the instructions for the basic clay mask recipe (see page 108). You may need to add an extra tablespoon of bottled or spring water, but do this carefully (a little at a time). Herbs are also sometimes available in capsule form. Use the contents of four capsules per mask and follow the basic recipe.

nuts and fruit

You can make masks and/or lotions using some of the fresh seasonal and all-year-round fruits available in your local supermarket. All of them are simple to make and fun to use. Several can be recommended for their excellent revitalizing, nourishing, and often astringent action on the skin, and a series of useful recipes is given below. Most are included in the six-week program. Follow the recommendations for your skin type.

If the consistency of your purée makes it difficult to work with, add a little white clay (see page 107) to thicken or live yogurt to thin. Use the tips of your fingers to apply the mask gently to your face and neck, starting from the center of the forehead and working outward. Work carefully around the eyes—none of these preparations must come into contact with them. Unless otherwise indicated, remove the mask using bottled or spring water or rosewater (see Hydrosols, page 126) and cotton balls.

almond

Almond nuts contain a variety of trace elements, vitamins A and B, and oleic acid. The mask can be used once a week for normal, dry, combination, or aging skin; the almond lotion (or milk) has a cleansing and nourishing action on normal, dry, or combination skin, and can be used daily for short periods.

TO MAKE A MASK
Crush ⅓ cup (50g.) peeled almonds in a mortar or blend in a food processor. Stir in about 3 tablespoons whole milk (a little at a time), enough to make a smooth paste that can be applied to the skin. Add, if you wish, one or two drops of rose attar (see page 62). Apply and leave on until dry (for about 30 minutes). Remove with cotton balls and bottled or spring water.

TO MAKE A LOTION
Dissolve ½ cup (50g.) peeled, finely crushed almonds—ground almonds save time but may not be so fresh—and 1fl. oz. (25g.) organic honey in 1pt. (500ml.) bottled or spring water, stir and leave to rest for 2 hours. Filter and keep in the coldest part of the refrigerator. Apply generously, twice daily, using cotton balls. Throw away any leftovers after a week.

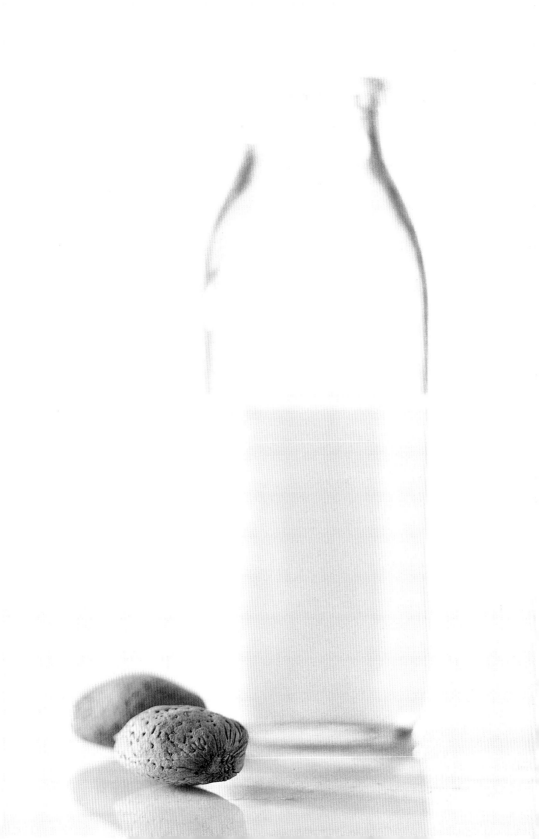

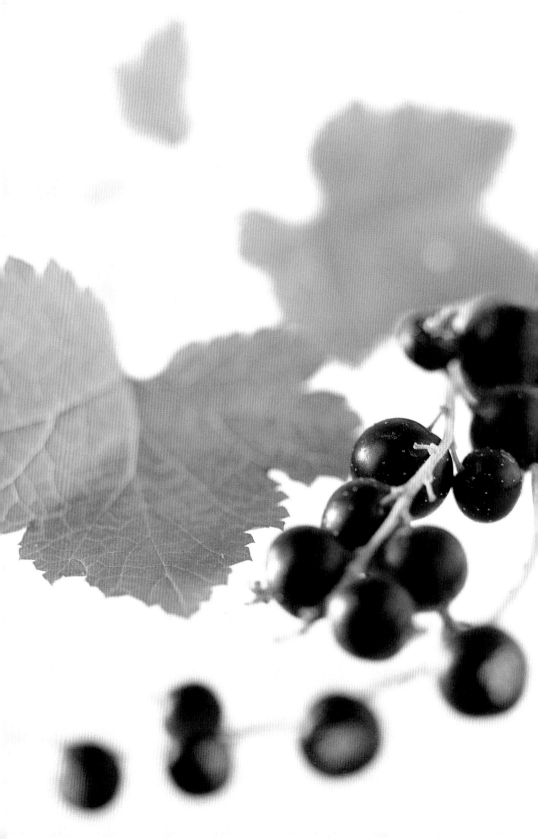

apricot

Fresh apricots are rich in vitamins A, B1, B2, and C, PP (a strong bactericide and astringent), and many important minerals (calcium, iron, magnesium, manganese, phosphorus, potassium, and sulfur). Applied twice a week, it is a good tonic for normal or dry skin.

TO MAKE A MASK

Peel and remove the stones from 2 ripe apricots. Crush with a fork or in a food processor and apply immediately to the skin. Leave on for 30 minutes, and then rinse off, using bottled or spring water or rosewater (see Hydrosols, page 126) and cotton balls.

avocado

Avocados are rich in amino acids and vitamins, and make excellent anti-aging masks for dry, combination, or mature skin.

TO MAKE A MASK

FOR DRY SKIN

Simply mash the flesh of 1 ripe avocado with a fork or in a food processor and apply immediately to the skin. Leave on for 30 minutes, and then rinse off with bottled or spring water or rosewater (see Hydrosols, page 126), using cotton balls.

For combination skin

Add 1 lightly beaten egg yolk to the mashed flesh of half an avocado and apply as above.

FOR AGING SKIN

As mask 2, stirring 1 tablespoon organic honey into the mix.

blackcurrant

This fruit makes an excellent tonic and hydrating mask for normal and dry skin and can be used twice a week. Blackcurrants are rich in trace elements, calcium, magnesium, potassium, vitamins B1, B2, B3, B5, B6, C, and flavonoids. After the mask, dab some almond lotion (see page 112) onto the skin with cotton balls to nourish.

TO MAKE A MASK

Using a fork, crush 3 tablespoons blackcurrants and mix with 2 tablespoons live yogurt. Apply to the skin and leave for 15 minutes. Rinse off with bottled or spring water, or rosewater (see Hydrosols, page 126), using cotton balls.

grape

Either color will do, but the juice must be freshly pressed. Like black-currants, grapes are rich in trace elements, calcium, magnesium, potassium, vitamins B_1, B_2, B_3, B_5, B_6, C, and flavonoids, but many of these are lost in the pasteurization process. Grape lotion can be used daily and is recommended for dry, aging and damaged skin.

TO MAKE A LOTION

It could hardly be simpler—just crush a few grapes, enough to make 2 tablespoons of juice, with a fork or in a blender, and filter. Apply the juice, using cotton balls. After 20 minutes, remove any stickiness with rosewater (see Hydrosols, page 126).

lemon

Lemons contain vitamins A, C, B_1, B_2 and B_3 or PP (a strong bactericide and astringent). They are good to use on oily skin, but the lotion given is adapted for the special needs of combination skin. It can be used once daily (unless otherwise indicated in the six-week plans, see pages 98–103). The quantity given is enough for a week.

TO MAKE A MASK

Add 1 teaspoon lemon juice to 1 stiffly beaten egg white. Apply to the skin and leave on for 10 minutes. Rinse off with bottled or spring water or rosewater (see Hydrosols, page 126).

TO MAKE A LOTION

Add 1 teaspoon lemon juice to 3½ fl.oz. (100ml.) rosewater (see Hydrosols, page 126) and 2 fl. oz. (approx. 50ml.) witch hazel (also see Hydrosols). Apply to the skin with cotton balls.

strawberry

This fruit contains salicylic acid, silica, and vitamins B, C, E, and K. Its astringent and revitalizing action is recommended for all skin types and can be used twice a week.

TO MAKE A MASK

Apply 2 tablespoons crushed strawberries to the skin and leave for 15 minutes. Rinse off with bottled or spring water or rosewater (see Hydrosols, page 126). For an even stronger toning effect, you can add 1 stiffly beaten egg white, 1 tablespoon rosewater (see Hydrosols), and 2 drops frankincense essential oil (see page 51) to the crushed fruit.

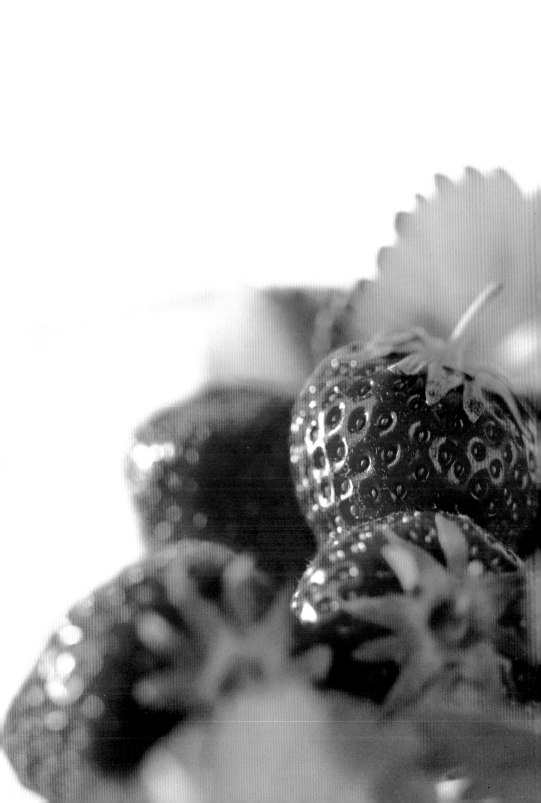

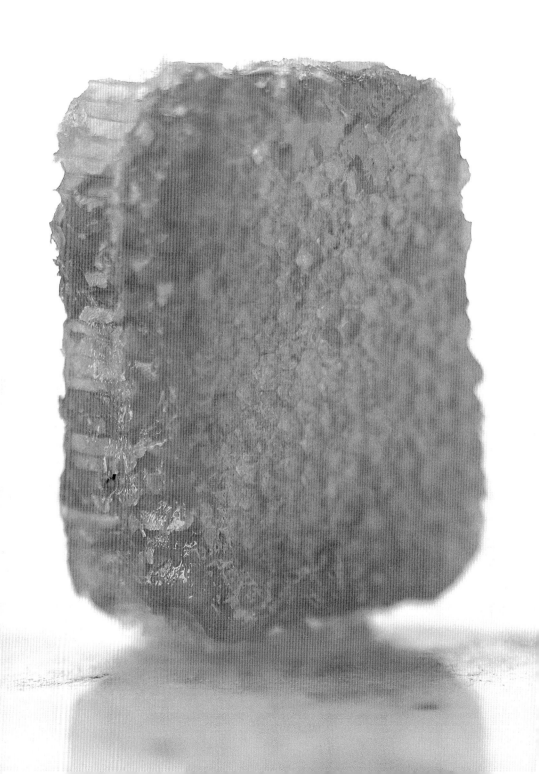

bee products

Among the natural ingredients beneficial to the skin, bee products are often neglected, although they have many advantages. They are inexpensive, are easily available in health stores and pharmacies, and work very well for wrinkles and damaged skin; they eliminate yeast and the microorganisms present in conditions such as acne and eczema.

honey

There are many valuable trace elements in organic honey that make it both nourishing and moisturizing for dry, tired skin—that is for skin dull or gray in appearance, cold to touch, and without much tone. However, it can be equally nourishing for normal skin. Honey also has useful antibacterial and fungicidal properties—hence the mask for oily or sensitive skin. Use once a week.

TO MAKE A MASK

FOR NORMAL SKIN
Mix 2½ fl.oz. (75ml.) organic live yogurt with 1 tablespoon fresh carrot juice, and add 1 tablespoon organic honey. If the mixture is too runny, and thus difficult to apply, thicken with 1 teaspoon white clay (see page 107). Apply to the skin and leave on for 20 minutes. Rinse off with bottled or spring water or rosewater (see Hydrosols, page 126). To adapt for dry or tired skin, add 1 tablespoon sweet almond carrier oil with the honey.

FOR DRY SKIN 1
Add 1 teaspoon organic honey and 1 teaspoon wheatgerm carrier oil to 2 tablespoons live yogurt, stirring well. Apply to the skin and leave on for 20 minutes. Rinse off, using bottled or spring water or rosewater (see Hydrosols, page 126) and cotton balls.

FOR DRY SKIN 2
Beat 1 egg white until stiff and then stir in 1 tablespoon organic honey, 1 tablespoon wheatgerm carrier oil, and 1 teaspoon lemon juice. Apply to the skin and leave for 20 minutes. Rinse off, using bottled or spring water, or rosewater (see Hydrosols, page 126) and cotton balls.

FOR OILY SKIN OR INFLAMMATION ON SENSITIVE SKIN

Peel a thick slice of cucumber—1 in. (2.5cm.) will be enough—and extract 1 tablespoon cucumber juice using a blender. Mix with 1 tablespoon honey and then add 1 tablespoon fresh whole milk and 1 tablespoon white or green clay (see page 107), stirring well. Apply to the skin and leave on for 20 minutes to remove impurities. Rinse off with bottled or spring water, or rosewater (see Hydrosols, page 126).

pollen

This bee product, available in a granular, unprocessed form, is rich in the amino acids, minerals, and vitamins needed for healthy skin and is especially useful for aging or devitalized skin types.

TO MAKE A MASK

Crush 1 heaping tablespoon unprocessed pollen in a blender and mix with 2 lightly beaten egg yolks. Apply to the face and neck, leave on for 30 minutes, and rinse off with bottled or spring water or rosewater (see Hydrosols, page 126). Use once or twice a week.

propolis

A wax produced by bees which acts as an antiseptic and fungicidal in the hives, propolis is available generally in liquid form from most health stores. Scientific studies have demonstrated its remarkable properties against a variety of microorganisms, especially yeast. Since these organisms are always present in oily skins, propolis is an effective way of readjusting the balance. In rare instances, some people develop a mild allergic reaction, so test first by applying a drop to your inner arm and checking for redness after a few minutes.

TO MAKE A MASK

Make a basic clay mask (see page 108). Add 1 teaspoon liquid propolis and 3 drops tea tree essential oil (see page 65), stirring well. Apply, leave until almost dry (30 minutes), and rinse off with bottled or spring water. Tone with a lotion of half rosewater and half witch hazel (see Hydrosols, page 126).

steaming

This is one of the simplest ways of deep-cleaning the skin. The traditional benefits of steaming, using just a bowl of boiling water, can be boosted by adding essential oil or herbs (dried or fresh) to the water.

On oily skin, steaming can be done once a week or every ten days, and for 6–8 minutes at a time. For combination skin, steaming for 5 minutes once a week is sufficient. Normal skin will benefit from steaming once every three weeks, as long as the exposure to steam is not prolonged (5 minutes should be your maximum). On dry or aging skin twice a month is the maximum, and for no more than 2 to 3 minutes at a time. Steaming is not recommended for extremely sensitive skin, severe inflammation, infection, sunburn, rosacea, or when many small blood vessels are apparent.

oils

Rose attar and niaouli are suitable for all skin types; for oily skin, choose chamomile; for dry skin, geranium; and for combination skin, lavender. You can treat infected acne with this method too, using 1–2 drops each of tea tree and lavender essential oil. After steaming as below, dry the skin lightly and then apply the same oils to the skin (diluted in a calendula carrier).

TO STEAM WITH OILS

Pour approx. 1 pt. (1 liter) boiling water into a large bowl and add 1–2 drops of your chosen oil. Place on a flat surface at a comfortable height, and sit before it with your face in the steam. Cover your head and the bowl with a towel. Once the treatment is over (see recommended times above), dry your face gently with cotton balls or a soft towel and tone with rosewater (see Hydrosols, page 126).

herbs

Lavender, marshmallow, and rosemary are all suitable for normal skin, as is a half-in-half mix of chamomile and rosemary. You can use lavender on dry skin, too. Several herbs are recommended for the treatment of inflammation, to kill bacteria or yeast, or to promote healing. The following are all good for oily skin, but, specifically, use chamomile or yarrow for inflamed skin, marigold for damaged skin, and thyme for infected skin. A half-in-half mix of chamomile and lavender is good for oily skin, too.

TO STEAM WITH HERBS

If you pour approx. 1pt. (1 liter) boiling water onto 1 tablespoon dried herbs or 2 tablespoons fresh herbs, you have an infusion with medicinal properties. Follow the method given for oils. If using chamomile, you can substitute a chamomile tea bag.

eating for healthy skin

Above a certain level of affluence in westernized countries we should not suffer from vitamin or mineral deficiencies, but in reality prolonged storage of fresh food in refrigerators reduces its nutritional value considerably. Fast and processed foods are also low in vitamins, and dieting is a common cause of deficiencies. Add to that the fact that stress and regular consumption of alcohol, tobacco, or recreational drugs tend to prevent the proper utilization of essential vitamins and minerals, and there is a heavy price to pay for the way we live our lives.

A varied diet, plus regular exercise, is one of the most important ways of looking young and healthy for a long time. The list that follows is a reminder of the vital ingredients necessary to combat the effects of time on your skin. Multivitamin and mineral supplements can play a supporting role in establishing a balanced diet.

Vitamin A (or retinol) A severe deficiency of vitamin A is rare, and taking excessive amounts of it may result in joint pain, scaling of the skin, and even birth defects. It is best absorbed in the form of betacarotene, which is found in vegetables. This group of pigments can be converted to vitamin A in the process of digestion, but it also has the capacity to absorb free radicals, an important factor in aging. Food sources: carrots, spinach, sweet potatoes, watercress, and dried apricots. Betacarotene can also be applied externally, as a cream for sensitive or aging skin.

Vitamin B_2 (or riboflavin) Minor deficiency causes seborrheic dermatitis or inflammation around the nose and mouth; a lack of B_2 is also associated with poor hair condition and nails that break easily. Food sources: wheatgerm, fortified breakfast cereals, milk, eggs, liver, and yeast extract.

Vitamin B_3 (or niacin) This vitamin reinforces the skin's natural protection against exposure to the sun, and deficiency can cause fatigue, depression, and dermatitis. Food sources: wheatgerm, brown rice, chicken, broccoli, and tuna.

Vitamin B_6 (or pyridoxine) A deficiency of vitamin B_6 causes excess sebum, resulting in an oily skin with inflammation, crusting, and scale. Food sources: wheatgerm, chicken, beef, yeast extract, and bananas.

Vitamin B_{12} A lack of B_{12} is common among vegetarians and vegans. Mild deficiency will cause fatigue and dry skin; a severe deficiency leads to anemia and

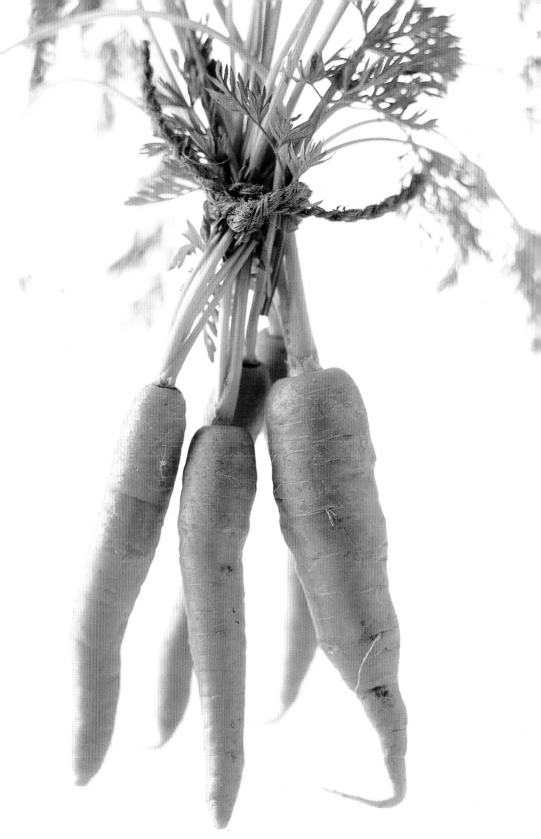

neurological damage. Food sources: red meat, liver, fish, and eggs.

Biotin Part of the vitamin B complex, biotin is known to have a direct action on oily skin. A lack of it is unusual in moderately affluent countries, but its manifestations are a fine scaly dermatitis or seborrheic dermatitis. Food sources: brewer's yeast, liver, kidney, wheat bran, and wheatgerm.

PABA (para-aminobenzoic or folic acid) Also part of the vitamin B complex, a deficiency of PABA results in skin conditions such as eczema and loss of pigmentation. Food sources: liver, brewer's yeast, wheatgerm, and molasses.

Vitamin C An important vitamin for the formation of collagen and for the healing of skin, vitamin C is not easily retained by the body. However, if it is taken along with bioflavonoids (or vitamin P), absorption is improved. Bioflavonoids are also useful for people with poor circulation or who bruise easily. Food sources: many raw fruits and vegetables, especially citrus fruits.

Vitamin D (or calciferol) Vegetarians, vegans, and lactating women are prone to calciferol deficiency, which may cause a weakening of the bones. Food sources: cod liver oil, fish, evaporated milk, and eggs.

Vitamin E (or tocoferol) This powerful antioxidant is the best friend of dry skin or of aging or menopausal skin made worse by poor circulation. Food sources: wheatgerm, safflower and sunflower oils, almonds, mayonnaise, and peanut butter.

Oleic, linoleic, and arachidonic acids (or vitamin F) These polyunsaturated fatty acids are crucially important for the vitality of the skin. Vitamin F represents 10 percent of the polyunsaturated fatty acids in the body, which is unable to synthesize them. Food sources: all the carrier oils that are listed on pages 41–47, but cold-pressed olive oil is probably the best.

Amino acids L-arginine and L-ornithine stimulate the formation of collagen and play an important role in healing; L-cysteine is also involved in the formation of collagen, as well as lessening the effects of smoking and radiation and promoting hair growth; L-lysine supports the immune system and is an effective treatment for cold sores. Food sources: red meat, milk, and nuts. They are also available in most health-food stores as food supplements.

Zinc Deficiency contributes to conditions such as eczema and acne and to poor nails. Food sources: cheese, whole-wheat bread, eggs, and chicken.

body pressure points

Stimulating acupressure points on the body is a useful and logical complement to the massage program on pages 70–97. You need to learn just a few extra points for an overall toning effect on blood circulation and the elimination of toxins, and to stimulate natural vitality and energy. Try to work on each of them once a day. They are all bilateral, so you need to stimulate each side of your body in turn. Rotate your index finger or thumb with firm pressure for about 1 minute at each point.

Point A: outside hand, between thumb and index finger Although it principally affects the upper part of the body and the face (in particular, each side of the nose), this point also has a direct effect on the large intestine. Its function is to aid the elimination of waste products and detoxification. It quickly begins to ache if massaged for too long.

Point B: end of elbow crease when arm folded across chest This enhances the action of A when used in association with it. The combination is also often effective in the treatment of hayfever, headache, colds, and rhinitis.

Point C: inner wrist, 2 thumbs' width from wrist crease, between tendons Well-known for its proven effect on travel sickness, morning sickness, and nausea induced by chemotherapy, this point, used in association with D, has a remarkably stimulating effect on the circulation of the blood, and a yin, cooling effect on the whole body. C and D are also a very effective combination for the relief of PMS and menstrual pain.

Point D: inside leg, 3 thumbs' width above ankle bone, on lower edge of tibia Its powerful balancing action and influence on the circulation of the blood throughout the body make this a valuable tool for general health.

Point E: just below knee, depression between bones, toward outside leg This has a beneficial effect on most of the face and is also a powerful point for the digestive system, for energizing the whole body, and for stimulating resistance to disease. For the face, use in association with A.

Point F: between first and second toe This point is a good energy regulator and very effective in reducing stress, especially if combined with C. Its action in helping the liver to detoxify the body makes it very important for acne, inflamed skin with pimples, and blackheads.

hydrosols

Otherwise known as hydrolats or floral waters, hydrosols are a liquid byproduct of the steam distillation process used to extract many essential oils. (They are not to be confused with flower waters, which are a mix of essential oil and purified water, plus a dispersing agent.)

A filtered mixture of the steaming water and the remaining active principles (in oil and plant form), hydrosols have similar properties to those essential oils, but a much gentler action. Their shelf life is limited, so suppliers often add potassium sorbate to extend their usefulness. They are an excellent way to tone, calm inflammations, or rebalance the skin.

Hydrosols, including rosewater and witch hazel, are available from some pharmacies and health stores; alternatively, you could try one of the mail-order sources listed here. (But make sure you are buying a hydrosol and not a flower water.) Rosemary hydrosol is particularly good for oily skin.

Hydrosols should be dabbed (not rubbed) onto the skin with cotton balls to create a thin film which can be quickly absorbed.

sources

⊠ Indicates that a mail-order service is available.

NEAL'S YARD REMEDIES ⊠
79 East Putnam Avenue
Greenwich, CT 06830
tel: 1-888-697-8721 (toll-free)
fax: 203-629-0886

CASWELL MASSEY ⊠
518 Lexington Avenue
New York, NY 10017
tel: 212-755-2254
fax: 212-777-4915

APHRODISIA ⊠
264 Bleecker Street
New York, NY 10014
tel: 212-989-6440
fax: 212-989-8027

LIBERTY NATURAL PRODUCTS ⊠
8120 SE Stark Street
Portland, OR 97215
tel: 800-289-8247
www.libertynatural.com

LEYDET AROMATICS ⊠
P. O. Box 2354
Fair Oaks, CA 95628
tel: 916-965-7546
www.leydet.com

EARTHBOUND ⊠
529 South Street
Philadelphia, PA 19147
tel: 215-627-1797
www.ebound.com

index

ACKNOWLEDGMENTS

Author acknowledgments My thanks to Sandra Beevor, Sally Chambers, Caroline Clayton, Zakia Collins, Maxine Harrison, Majken Kruse, Jane Lewis, Dee Markham, Sandra Saunders, and Tina Stevens, who participated in the trials. Special thanks to Shirley and Len Price for reading and commenting on the manuscript.

Picture credits The massage photographs were taken by Maureen Barrymore; participants in the trials were photographed by James Darrell; and the photographs of flowers, herbs, and recipe ingredients were taken by Diana Miller and styled by Wei Tang. The acupressure photograph on page 26 was taken by Sandra Lousada/Collections.

The mission of Storey Communications is to serve our customers by publishing practical information that encourages personal independence in harmony with the environment.

United States edition published in 2000 by Storey Books, Schoolhouse Road, Pownal, Vermont 05261

United Kingdom edition published in 1999 by Quadrille Publishing Limited, Alhambra House, 27-31 Charing Cross Road, London, WC2H 0LS

Publishing Director: Anne Furniss
Creative Director: Mary Evans
Consultant Art Director: Helen Lewis
Art Editor: Rachel Gibson
Editor: Mary Davies
Production: Vincent Smith, Candida Jackson

This publication is intended to provide educational information for the reader on the covered subject. It is not intended to take the place of personalized medical counseling, diagnosis, and treatment from a trained health professional.

Printed and bound in Hong Kong
10 9 8 7 6 5 4 3 2 1
ISBN 1-58017-242-3

Library of Congress Cataloging-in-Publication Data
Cousin, Pierre Jean.
    Facelift at your fingertips: an aromathreapy massage program for healthy skin and a younger face / Pierre Jean Cousin.—U.S. ed.
        p. cm.
    U.K. ed. pub. with title: Facelift at your fingertips. London : Quadrille Pub., 1999.
    Includes index.
    ISBN 1-58017-242-3 (pbk. : alk.paper)
    1. Aromatherapy massage. 2. Skin—Care and hygiene.
3. Essences and essential oils. 4. Beauty, Personal.
5. Women—Health and hygiene. I. Title.
RM666.A68 C68 2000
646.7'26—dc21
                                                                99-046586